◆

# Posttraumatic Stress Disorder: DSM-IV and Beyond

◆

◆

# Posttraumatic Stress Disorder: DSM-IV and Beyond

◆

Edited by

**Jonathan R. T. Davidson, M.D.**
Associate Professor and Director,
  Anxiety and Traumatic Stress Program
Department of Psychiatry
Duke University Medical Center
Durham, North Carolina

**Edna B. Foa, Ph.D.**
Professor of Psychiatry and Director,
  Anxiety Disorders Clinic
Medical College of Pennsylvania
Philadelphia, Pennsylvania

Washington, DC
London, England

**Note:** The authors have worked to ensure that all information in the book concerning drug dosages, schedules, and routes of administration is accurate as of the time of publication and consistent with standards set by the U.S. Food and Drug Administration and the general medical community. As medical research and practice advance, however, therapeutic standards may change. For this reason and because human and mechanical errors sometimes occur, we recommend that readers follow the advice of a physician who is directly involved in their care or the care of a member of their family.

This book covers many major issues regarding PTSD but does not address other important topics (e.g., treatment or cross-cultural aspects of the disorder). Also, this book should not be construed as an extended DSM report on PTSD, nor will all of its recommendations be incorporated into the DSM-IV manual. Such decisions are based on the consideration of many factors, some of which are beyond the scope of this book. The views expressed here are those of the authors and do not represent the official positions of the DSM-IV Task Force, the American Psychiatric Press, or the American Psychiatric Association.

American Psychiatric Press, Inc.
1400 K Street, N.W., Washington, DC 20005

**Library of Congress Cataloging-in-Publication Data**
Posttraumatic stress disorder: DSM-IV and Beyond / [edited by]
    Jonathan R.T. Davidson, Edna B. Foa.
        p. cm.
    Includes bibliographical references and index.
    ISBN 0-88048-502-7 (alk. paper)
    1. Post-traumatic stress disorder. 2. Diagnostic and statistical
manual of mental disorders. I. Davidson, Jonathan R. T., 1943–
II. Foa, Edna B.
    [DNLM: 1. Stress Disorders, Post-Traumatic. 2. Stress Disorders,
    Post-Traumatic—classification. WM 170 P8575]
    RC552.P678679    1992
    616.85'21—dc20                                          92-7052
                                                            CIP
**British Library Cataloging in Publication Data**
A CIP record is available from the British Library.

# Table of Contents

## Section IV: Classification of Posttraumatic Stress Disorder

## Section V: Posttraumatic Stress Disorder in Relation to Other Disorders

## Appendixes

# Contributors

**Arthur S. Blank, Jr., M.D.**
Director of Readjustment Counseling Service, Department of Medicine and Surgery, Veterans Administration, Washington, DC

**Elizabeth A. Brett, Ph.D.**
Associate Clinical Professor of Psychiatry and Psychology, Yale University School of Medicine, New Haven, Connecticut

**Jonathan R. T. Davidson, M.D.**
Associate Professor and Director, Anxiety and Traumatic Stress Program, Department of Psychiatry, Duke University Medical Center, Durham, North Carolina

**John A. Fairbank, Ph.D.**
Senior Research Clinical Psychologist, Center for Social Research and Policy Analysis, Research Triangle Institute, Research Triangle Park, North Carolina

**Edna B. Foa, Ph.D.**
Professor of Psychiatry and Director, Anxiety Disorders Clinic, Medical College of Pennsylvania, Philadelphia, Pennsylvania

**Bonnie L. Green, Ph.D.**
Associate Professor of Psychiatry, Department of Psychiatry, George Washington University Medical School, Washington, DC

**Judith L. Herman, M.D.**
Associate Clinical Professor of Psychiatry, Harvard Medical School, Boston, Massachusetts; Cambridge Hospital, Cambridge, Massachusetts

**Terence M. Keane, Ph.D.**
Chief of Psychology and Director, Behavioral Science Division, National Center for Posttraumatic Stress Disorder, Boston, Massachusetts; Veterans Administration Medical Center, Boston, Massachusetts; Department of Psychology, Tufts—New England Medical Center, Boston, Massachusetts

**Dean G. Kilpatrick, Ph.D.**
Director, Crime Victims Research and Treatment Center, Department

of Psychiatry and Behavioral Sciences, Medical University of South Carolina, Charleston, South Carolina

**John S. March, M.D., M.P.H.**
Associate Professor of Psychiatry, Department of Psychiatry, Duke University Medical Center, Durham, North Carolina

**Richard J. McNally, Ph.D.**
Associate Professor, Department of Psychology, Harvard University, Cambridge, Massachusetts

**Barbara Olasov Rothbaum, Ph.D.**
Assistant Professor, Department of Psychiatry, The Emory Clinic, Section of Psychiatry, Atlanta, Georgia

**Roger K. Pitman, M.D.**
Clinical Investigator, Veterans Administration Medical Center, Manchester, New Hampshire; Associate Professor of Psychiatry, Harvard Medical School, Boston, Massachusetts

**Heidi S. Resnick, Ph.D.**
Assistant Professor, Department of Psychiatry and Behavioral Sciences, Crime Victims Research and Treatment Center, Medical University of South Carolina, Charleston, South Carolina

**Philip A. Saigh, Ph.D.**
Professor, Graduate School and University Center, City University of New York, New York, New York

# Introduction

Traumatic neuroses is a convenient term, but . . . it is apt to include far too much . . . in a so called traumatic neurosis we may have to deal with an organic nerve injury, with hysteria, the result of injury, with shock . . . with neurasthenia, or even with a true psychosis. (Lancet 1891, p. 160)

Posttraumatic stress disorder (PTSD) has come of age. It was formally recognized and codified in DSM-III (American Psychiatric Association 1980). This disorder has a long tradition, having been described in association with battle and masquerading under a variety of names. Many of these names highlighted certain aspects of the disorder, such as cardiac symptoms ("soldier's heart"), exhaustion ("battle fatigue"), neurotic manifestations ("combat neurosis") and "traumatic neurosis" to refer to the singular link with a traumatic event. For the most part, at least historically, interest in traumatic disorders waxed around wartime and waned during peace. As an example, DSM-I, which was published after World War II (American Psychiatric Association 1952), not only recognized traumatic neurosis but gave it a deserved emphasis in the nomenclature, and provided two subtypes. DSM-II, on the other hand, which was published more than 20 years after the end of World War II but before Vietnam (American Psychiatric Association 1968), relegated trauma-related disorders to just one example of situational disturbances of adult life, equating it with the Ganser syndrome and resentment associated with unwanted pregnancy. It is now recognized that PTSD does not belong to wartime alone, but may also arise from a variety of traumatic events that can occur throughout the life cycle to both men and women. It is estimated that 4 out of 10 Americans have experienced major trauma, and the disorder may be present in 9% of the population in the United States (Breslau et al. 1991). To underscore the heavy individual and societal cost of PTSD, we may refer to epidemiological data that find a 19% risk of suicide attempts in individuals who, for the most part, had neither received treatment nor were aware of their PTSD. There is also an increased risk of associated chronic medical disorders such as hypertension, bronchial asthma, and peptic ulcer, as well as a variety of psychological disorders (Davidson et al. 1991).

Having established the magnitude and cost of PTSD, what are some of the major questions that we must address, and what contributions might be made by this book, whose subject is the diagnosis of PTSD? First, a brief word about the origin of this volume, which arose from the revision process for the forthcoming *Diagnostic and Statistical Manual of Mental Disorders, 4th Edition* (DSM-IV): all the chapters are written by members of the sub-workgroup on PTSD for DSM-IV. In fulfilling its charge, the committee members identified a number of key questions concerning the diagnosis of PTSD that they thought should be addressed by DSM-IV, and, more importantly, that have broad relevance to PTSD as a whole. These can be grouped into five main areas:

1. Specifying the clinical phenomenology (i.e., course, duration, subtypes) and the nature of the stressor criteria (what it is that makes an event traumatic);
2. Studying specific victim groups with a goal to establishing cohesiveness of the syndrome;
3. Considering the prevalence, characteristics, and risk factors of PTSD in the community as a whole and among at-risk epidemiological groups;
4. Considering where and how PTSD should be classified: whether by etiology, pathophysiology, or symptomatology; and
5. Examining the relationship of PTSD to other disorders. This includes boundary issues with related disorders, and the notion that several traumatic disorders may exist, including one particular symptom constellation following prolonged and repeated victimization.

Among the unresolved clinical questions is the longitudinal course of PTSD and its relationship to subtyping of the disorders. These are discussed in chapters by Blank (Chapter 1) and by Rothbaum and Foa (Chapter 2). As currently formulated in DSM-III-R (American Psychiatric Association 1987), PTSD must be present for at least 1 month for the diagnosis to be made. Based on the finding that many rape victims with PTSD achieve spontaneous recovery during the first 3 months (Rothbaum et al., in press), Rothbaum and Foa discuss whether a 3-month cutoff point would be a more appropriate minimum duration than the 1-month period that is currently required. Both chapters illuminate the important question of normal versus abnormal responses to trauma.

March (Chapter 3) addresses the crucial question of the traumatic event (i.e., Criterion A of the diagnostic criteria). Because this criterion serves as a gatekeeper, its definition is of fundamental importance: a broad definition will open up the diagnosis of PTSD to many victims of stressful events, whereas a narrow definition will limit the prevalence of this disorder. The impact of the stressful event on an individual is affected both by characteristics of the event and by appraisal or subjective reaction by the person experiencing it. March discusses the importance of both factors as they influence the risk for developing PTSD. In a later chapter, Kilpatrick and Resnick (Chapter 7) also discuss the factors of the traumatic event that increase the risk of PTSD.

In the second section of this book, four chapters survey the literature on PTSD in various populations including children, victims of disaster, Vietnam combat veterans, and victims of crime. The authors of all four chapters agree with the basic validity of the current symptom criteria for PTSD and conclude that no major changes are necessary in this respect. The authors find validation of the DSM-III criteria by means of factor analysis, frequency counts, and internal consistency of the three criteria clusters: reexperiencing, avoidance, and arousal. McNally (Chapter 4) concludes that the criteria clusters, in general, are appropriate to traumatized children. Green, Keane, and Kilpatrick and Resnick (Chapters 5, 6, and 7) note a major weakness of the current criteria in their handling of the avoidant symptoms. It is possible that the minimum requirement of three avoidance symptoms is too high and that a distinction should be made between those avoidant symptoms that are specific to PTSD and those that are common to other disorders as well. Kilpatrick and Resnick present interesting analysis on the effect of altering the required minimum number of avoidant symptoms upon community prevalence rates of PTSD.

Much has been learned in recent years about the epidemiology of PTSD, with all studies indicating it to be a problem of substantial magnitude in the general population. A number of epidemiological risk factors have been identified, strongly suggesting the importance of genetic influence, early adverse experiences in childhood, personality factors, and physical harm. These are reviewed by Davidson and Fairbank (Chapter 8), who conclude that PTSD deserves separate classification on the basis of etiology, rather than its preservation as an anxiety disorder.

The issue of classification is formally addressed by Pitman (Chapter 9), who points out that classifications of illness have historically followed a hierarchy of increasing desirability. At the lowest end is classification by symptomatology, followed by structural change, pathogenesis, and, ultimately, by etiology. Currently questions in regard of clarifying PTSD include whether we have we yet reached the point at which we can argue for an etiologically based classification. This would mean the creation of a separate category of stressor of trauma-related psychological disorders, of which PTSD would serve as a standard bearer with others presumably in tow. Do we yet know enough about the etiology of PTSD? Is the case for retaining PTSD as a pathological form of anxiety more compelling? There is also some basis for regarding PTSD as a pathological state of dissociation, in which case it might properly belong among the dissociative disorders. These issues are concisely addressed by Pitman as well as Brett (Chapter 10).

The boundary issue between PTSD and simple phobia following a traumatic event is addressed by McNally and by Saigh (Chapter 11). The notion of other posttraumatic syndromes is discussed by Herman in her review of the literature concerning sequelae of prolonged and repeated interpersonal trauma. She notes that such prolonged trauma produces a constellation of affective, somatic, and dissociative symptoms, accompanied by identity problems, pathological relationships, and repeated self-injurious behavior. Herman proposes calling this syndrome "disorders of extreme stress not otherwise specified" (DESNOS).

In summary, our objective for this volume is to present critical summaries of the literature on the following issues: longitudinal course, subtypes and outcome; the nature of the traumatic event ("the stressor"); the symptom picture in different victim groups; risk factors and community prevalence; the neurobiology of PTSD; classification; boundary questions regarding PTSD, simple phobia, dissociative disorders, and anxiety; and the possible existence of a new class of traumatic stress syndromes that may not be adequately accounted for within the current framework of PTSD.

All chapters follow a standard methodology and include information obtained by computer-based literature searches, unpublished data on ongoing studies, and presentation at meetings. Key words were used for each literature search as appropriate. In general, literature was limited to the post–1980 era (i.e., DSM-III and DSM-III-R) and the use of structured or standard diagnostic interviews were usually required, but this was not invariably the case.

The chapters are based on the reviews submitted to the DSM-IV Committee, but their content and conclusions are addressed to a wider audience than those who are merely concerned with the DSM-IV. We discuss their implications in an epilogue. In addition, we provide a brief summary of each chapter.

Jonathan R. T. Davidson, M.D.
Edna B. Foa, Ph.D.

# References

American Psychiatric Association: Diagnostic and Statistical Manual: Mental Disorders. Washington, DC, American Psychiatric Association, 1952

American Psychiatric Association: Diagnostic and Statistical Manual of Mental Disorders, 2nd Edition. Washington, DC, American Psychiatric Association, 1968

American Psychiatric Association: Diagnostic and Statistical Manual of Mental Disorders, 3rd Edition. Washington, DC, American Psychiatric Association, 1980

American Psychiatric Association: Diagnostic and Statistical Manual of Mental Disorders, 3rd Edition, Revised. Washington, DC, American Psychiatric Association, 1987

Breslau N, Davis GC, Andreski P: Traumatic events and post-traumatic stress disorder in an urban population of young adults. Arch Gen Psychiatry 48:216–222, 1991

Davidson JRT, Hughes DL, Blazer DG, et al: Posttraumatic stress disorder in the community: an epidemiological study. Psychol Med 2:713–721, 1991

Rothbaum BO, Foa EB, Riggs DR, et al: A prospective examination of post-traumatic stress disorder in rape victims. Journal of Traumatic Stress (in press)

◆

# Section I:

# Clinical Phenomenology: Course, Subtypes, and Trauma

◆

# ◆ 1 ◆ The Longitudinal Course of Posttraumatic Stress Disorder

Arthur S. Blank, Jr., M.D.

**Summary**　　　　In this chapter, the author reviews the natural history of posttraumatic stress disorder (PTSD) over time, with respect to symptom onset, course, and type; the existence of subclinical PTSD is also discussed. Differential variation of intrusive and avoidant PTSD symptoms are then described. Numerous factors can influence course, and these are identified. The effect of secondary gain is assessed. Finally, the author critically addresses methodological variables that can affect research findings.

## Introduction and Background

This chapter concerns the time dimension or natural history of PTSD, as reflected in recent published literature. Case-oriented literature prior to 1980, stretching back to early psychoanalytic writings on traumatic war neurosis in World War I veterans, provides some information about longitudinal course. However, that information was not significantly tapped by *Diagnostic and Statistical Manual of Mental Disorders, 3rd Edition* (DSM-III; American Psychiatric Association 1980) and *3rd Edition, Revised* (DSM-III-R; American Psychiatric Association 1987), possibly because of the high priority need for establishing (DSM-III) and refining (DSM-III-R) cross-sectional descriptive criteria. Thus, DSM-III-R says about course and subtypes only that "Symptoms usually begin immediately or soon after the trauma. Reexperiencing symptoms may develop after a latency period of months or years following the trauma, though avoidance symptoms have usually been present during this period" (p. 249).

3

The purpose of the following review is to ascertain what information is available especially from the post–1980 period about longitudinal course. After a statement of key issues, I describe the scope and method of the review, summarize published findings, and indicate problems and challenges concerning this topic. Although my discussion in this chapter emphasizes literature on the longitudinal course of PTSD, it also addresses issues of subtype and early remission that are developed further in Chapter 2 by Rothbaum and Foa. Suggested recommendations for *Diagnostic and Statistical Manual of Mental Disorders, 4th Edition* (DSM-IV) are presented separately in Appendix 1.

# Statement of the Issue

◆ What is the longitudinal course of PTSD?
◆ What are typical patterns with respect to longitudinal course, such as acute, chronic, delayed, intermittent or recurrent, reactivated, and residual?
◆ Is there a posttraumatic stress reaction of a V code nature (i.e., a "normal" posttraumatic stress reaction distinguishable either in course, or otherwise, from PTSD)?
◆ Aside from patterns of onset or duration, how do symptoms vary over time, especially with reference to the DSM-III-R categories of intrusion, avoidance, and hyperarousal?
◆ How does type of trauma affect course?
◆ What factors may be associated with exacerbation or amelioration during the course of the disorder?
◆ What are the effects, on course, of secondary gain, and what are the effects of the disorder over time on functioning?
◆ What are some limitations of recently published studies, and what are key problems in the investigation (including measurement) of longitudinal course?

# Method and Scope

A computer search of PTSD literature covering the years 1970 to 1989 using key terms such as "course," "longitudinal course," "follow-up," and "outcome," was obtained. In addition, the author used a personal collection of papers plus others furnished by DSM-IV PTSD Committee members, and by staff of the Department of Veterans Affairs Vietnam Veterans Counseling and Outreach Centers. Additional papers were obtained from various authors.

The number of reports that formally study the longitudinal course of PTSD is small. Therefore, a wide range of reports that might possibly contain information about course were reviewed. Included in the review were those papers that either contain a reasonably valid and explicit determination of PTSD case-ness, or data from which PTSD can be fairly well inferred.

For the most part, literature concerning the outcome of sexual or physical abuse in childhood, such as multiple personality disorder, was not included. Although these outcomes are probably related to traumatic stress and are at least closely related to PTSD, it appeared that their published literature does not yet clarify relationship to PTSD in a way that will contribute to a statement concerning course. Also not included are some otherwise valuable studies where the relationship of the symptoms described in DSM-III-R to PTSD could not be sufficiently determined for purposes of this chapter.

In general, my focus is on studies that treat the manifestations of PTSD over time. Because only three authors or groups of authors have utilized repeated measures, a number of long-term follow-up studies with one-point measures have been included.

Studies were catalogued (see Table 1–1) with respect to time from trauma to point of subject evaluation, diagnostic criteria and method used, use (or nonuse) of repeated measures, type of sample, number of subjects, type of trauma, mean age of subjects, ratio of males to females, and typical response rate.

## Aggregate Summary of Findings

### PTSD's Longitudinal Course

Consistent with the earlier clinical case literature on traumatic neurosis, most studies have found that PTSD often persists over time, or occurs long after the trauma. This is especially so if the trauma has been pro-

**Table 1–1.**   Studies evaluating the manifestations of PTSD over time

| Author(s) | Duration | Crit | Diagnostic Method | Reported Measures | Sample Type | N | Trauma Type | Mean Age | % M/F | Typical Response Rate |
|---|---|---|---|---|---|---|---|---|---|---|
| Archibald and Tuddenham 1965 | 20+ yrs | GS | CL;Q | No | Clin | 157 | War | 45 (est.) | 100/0 | ? |
| Goldstein et al. 1987 | 40 yrs | III | CSSI | No | Fol-Up | 41 | POW | 65 | 100/0 | ? |
| Goodwin 1985 | 1 wk to 24 yrs | III | CL | No | Case | 3 | Incest | a) 2 b) 14 c) 28 | 0/100 | N/A |
| Green et al. 1990 | 12 yrs | III-R | PEF; SCID; SCL-90 | Yes | Cmty | 120 | Flood | 53.5 | 38/62 | 39% |
| Kilpatrick et al. 1987 | 15 yrs (mean) | III | DIS by clinician | No | Cmty | 391 | Crime | 39.8 | 0/100 | 42.8% |
| Kluznik et al. 1986 | 40 yrs | III | CSI; Psych. HX | No | Fol-Up | 188 | POW | 65 | 100/0 | 53% |
| Kulka et al. 1990 | 19 yrs | III-R | MPTSD | No | Cmty | 3700 | War | 43 (est. av.) | 99.8/0.2 | 80% |
| McFarlane 1986a | 29 mos | III | Q (GHQ) | Yes | Cmty | 469 | Nat Dis | 36 | ? | 80% |
| McFarlane 1986b | 2 wks to 30 mos | III | CL | No | Case | 36 | Nat Dis | 35 | 46/64 | N/A |
| McFarlane 1987 | 26 mos | III | Q | Yes | Cmty | 808 | Nat Dis | 8.2 | 53/47 | 52% |
| McFarlane et al. 1987 | 26 mos | III | Q | Yes | Cmty | 808 | Nat Dis | 8.2 | 53/47 | 52% |
| McFarlane 1988a | 3.5 yrs | III | CSI; DIS | Yes | Cmty | 50 | Nat Dis | ? | ? | 85% |
| McFarlane 1988b | 29 mos | III | Q (CHQ, IES) | Yes | Cmty | 469 | Nat Dis | 36 | ? | 67% |
| McFarlane (pers. comm., August 1989) | 3.5 yrs | III | CSI-DIS; Q (GHQ) | Yes | Cmty | 147 of 469 | Nat Dis | ? | ? | 86% |

| Study | Duration | Crit | Diagnostic Method | | Sample Type | N | Trauma Type | Age | Sex | % |
|---|---|---|---|---|---|---|---|---|---|---|
| McFarlane 1989 | 29 mos | III | Q (GHQ) | Yes | Cmty | 469 | Nat Dis | 36 | ? | 72% |
| Saigh 1988 | 10.5 mos | III | CSI | No | Cmty | 12 | War | 21 (est) | 0/100 | 92% |
| Solomon et al. 1987a | 3 yrs | III | Clinical Records | No | Clin | 35 | War | 31 | 100/0 | N/A |
| Solomon 1987 | 2 yrs | III | CL;Q;IES | No | Clin, Cmty | 588 | War | ? | 100/0 | ? |
| Solomon and Mikulincer 1987 | 1 yr | III | CL;Q;IES | No | Cmty, Clin | 804* | War | 28.5 | 100/0 | 82% |
| Solomon et al. 1987b | 1 yr | III | CL;Q;IES | No | Clin | 382* | War | 28.5 | 100/0 | 82% |
| Solomon et al. 1987c | 1 yr | III | CL;Q;IES | No | Clin, Cmty | 716* | War | 28.5 | 100/0 | 81% |
| Solomon et al. 1988a | 1 yr | III | CL;CSSI; SCL-90;Q | No | Clin | 104* | War | 30 | 100/0 | ? |
| Solomon and Mikulincer 1988 | 2 yrs | III | IES;Q | Yes | Clin; Cmty | 483* | War | 28.5 | 100/0 | 75% |
| Solomon et al. 1988b | 3 yrs | III | Q | Yes | Clin | 262* | War | 29 | 100/0 | 71% |
| Solomon et al. 1988c | 2 yrs | III | Q | Yes | Clin | 382* | War | 28.5 | 100/0 | 82% |
| Solomon 1989b | 3 yrs | III | IES;Q | Yes | Clin | 329* | War | 28.5 | 100/0 | 46% |
| Solomon et al. 1989 | 6 yrs | III | Psych Hx | No | Clin | 150 | War | 29 | 100/0 | N/A |
| Speed et al. 1989 | 40+ yrs | III | CL;CSI | No | Fol-Up | 62 (est) | POW | 65 | 100/0 | N/A |
| Terr 1983 | 4 yrs | III | CL | Yes | Clin | 26 | Kidnapped & buried children | ? | ? | N/A |
| Zeiss and Dickman 1989 | 40 yrs | III | Q | No | Fol-Up | 442 | POW | 63.7 | ? | 44% |

*Sample overlaps with that of Solomon et al. 1987b. *Duration:* Length of time from trauma to study. *Crit:* Diagnostic criteria (DSM-III; DSM-III-R, GS—Gross Stress Reaction). *Diagnostic Method:* Psych. Hx—Psychiatric History; CL—Clinical interview; CSI—Structured interview, clinician; CSSI—Semistructured interview, clinician; MPTSD—Mississippi PTSD scale; Q—self-report questionnaire, IES—Impact of Events Scale; DIS—Diagnostic Interview Schedule; SCID—Structured Clinical Interview DSM-III-R; SCL-90—Symptom Checklist-90. *Sample Type:* Case; Clin—Clinical; Cmty—Community; Fol-Up—Follow-up, invited for an exam. *Trauma Type:* War; Nat Dis—Natural disaster; Crime. N/A: Not applicable. *III:* DSM-III. *III-R:* DSM-III-R. Unless otherwise specified (MPTSD, DIS, SCID), the PTSD instrument utilized in interviews was of *ad hoc* design based on the Dx criteria shown. Identical *N*s indicate multiple reports on same sample.

longed and complex, as in the instances of wartime combat and prisoner of war (POW) incarceration, but this also may be the case when the trauma is of relatively short duration. For example, in the largest epidemiologic study on PTSD to date, Kulka and colleagues (1990) found a 1987–1988 PTSD prevalence rate of 15% in Vietnam veterans (projectable to the entire community population of 3.14 million) approximately 19 years, on the average, after war zone traumatic stress.

Further, Goldstein and colleagues (1987) found a current prevalence of 50% and Kluznik and colleagues (1986) a current prevalence of 47% in former World War II POWs approximately 40 years after combat duty and prison camp confinement. McFarlane (1986a) found that 14% of a community sample of disaster survivors (brushfire fighters; duration of traumatic stress averaged approximately 16 hours) showed PTSD at 29 months follow-up. Solomon (1987) found that 56% of 3,553 Israeli soldiers who had had acute combat stress reaction during the 1982 Lebanon War showed PTSD at 2 years follow-up, and that 18% of 236 combat soldiers who had not had combat stress reaction also showed PTSD at the 2-year follow-up point.

All these studies confirm the earlier findings of Archibald and Tuddenham (1965), who reported in 1965 on a 20-year follow-up of 77 World War II and Korean War veterans with persisting poststress or gross stress syndrome, at least half of whom would probably qualify for the current diagnosis of PTSD.

In a community sample of 391 adult females, of whom 295 had been victimized by some type of crime, Kilpatrick and colleagues (1987) found that the lifetime rate of PTSD postcrime was 27.8% with a current prevalence of 7.5%. This was with an average time elapsed, since the criminal assault, of 15 years.

## Variations in Course in Relation to Other Aspects of PTSD

There are multiple variations in the natural history of PTSD, and there is evidence to suggest discrimination among acute, delayed, chronic, intermittent, residual, and reactivated patterns. Longitudinal data on survivors of varying types of traumatic stress also justify the establishment of a posttraumatic stress syndrome where full diagnostic criteria are not met.

### Australian Studies

In a report of 36 Australian brush firefighters, all of whom he saw clinically, McFarlane (1986b) reported that the first cases of acute PTSD presented for treatment at 1 to 4 months posttrauma, chronic cases presented at 10 to 20 months (although the onset of symptoms may have been earlier), and three cases showed a delayed onset 16 to 18 months posttrauma triggered by further stressful experiences.

Evidence for both the delayed emergence of PTSD and for the resolution of chronic cases is contained in McFarlane's 1986 report (1986a) on 469 brushfire fighters. At 11 months posttrauma, PTSD had emerged in 41 cases and resolved in 59 cases. At 29 months follow-up, PTSD had emerged in another 52 cases but had resolved in another 35. Only 53% of those who showed PTSD at 4 months also showed it at 29 months. McFarlane thereupon proposed three subtypes of PTSD: chronic, recurrent, and delayed onset.

In his study of 808 schoolchildren exposed to the same 1983 Australian brushfire, McFarlane (1987; McFarlane et al. 1987), while presenting data only on posttraumatic symptoms and not clearly establishing case-ness, probably demonstrates that, with measures at 2, 8, and 26 months, there were few cases before 2 months, and little diminution in cases over time up to the 29-month point.

In a further report on the 469 brushfire fighters, McFarlane (1988b) extracted a random subsample of 50 subjects from a subsample of 351 identified as at high risk for PTSD. Those subjects were measured at 4, 8, 11, 29, and 42 months (with shrinkage from $n = 50$ at 8 months to $n = 34$ at 42 months). In this particular trauma group, McFarlane found variations in diagnostic sensitivity and specificity of intrusion, avoidance, and hyperarousal symptoms, both cross-sectionally and over time, and suggested that intrusion symptoms may be more prominent early in the disorder and then fade over time. In this report he added "borderline chronic" to a list of possible variations, in that some subjects with subthreshold symptoms at one point in time later fully qualified for the diagnosis.

Overall, these and other of McFarlane's reports (1988b, 1989) document that PTSD may have either an acute or delayed onset and then remit or persist as a chronic form, which in turn may resolve, recur, or fluctuate in intensity.

Although these findings emerge from a population exposed to only one particular set of traumatic stressors, it is my assessment that a similar range of longitudinal course patterns is present for PTSD generally, particularly in light of the fact that the same patterns have been seen clinically in veterans of the Vietnam War over the past 20 years.

### Israeli Studies

Several reports by Solomon and colleagues on Israeli combat soldiers shed light on the course of PTSD. Although data were obtained only from psychiatric records, Solomon's 1987 study of 35 soldiers with multiple episodes of PTSD is useful (Solomon et al. 1987a). Of the 35 cases, 8 showed "uncomplicated reactivation" of PTSD. That is, these subjects had had a previous episode of PTSD followed by a full clearing of symptoms, but then they had developed acute PTSD in response to subsequent combat stress. Twenty-seven others in the group of 35 first had an episode of combat stress reaction (CSR), which may or may not have consisted of PTSD, and then were left with heightened vulnerability. Eighteen of these had a specific sensitivity—that is, some degree of exacerbation of PTSD symptoms on exposure to specific combat-related stimuli; 3 in the group displayed acute symptoms in response to stimuli that were only distantly related to the original trauma; and a final 6 subjects had chronic PTSD.

One contribution of this report is its formulation of the concept of "reactivated" PTSD. However, the report does not rule out the alternate hypothesis that the second discrete episode of PTSD was largely independent of the first episode (i.e., it would have occurred in the same individual in response to the second episode of traumatic stressors, even if the first episode of PTSD had not occurred).

Further reports by Solomon and colleagues have been based on large (e.g., $N = 382$) samples of Israeli combat soldiers, and various controls. These reports (Solomon 1987, 1989a; Solomon and Mikulincer 1987, 1988; Solomon et al. 1987b, 1987c, 1988a, 1988b, 1988c, 1989) reveal:

◆ Combat soldiers may show acute combat stress reaction, which is labile and more polymorphous than PTSD, and includes restlessness, psychomotor retardation, withdrawal, sympathetic hyperactivity, hyperstartle, confusion, nausea and vomiting, and paranoid reactions. Elsewhere, Rahe (1988) also includes, as possible features of acute stress reaction, overwhelming fear, reluctance to leave a secure setting, seizures, or paralysis. This acute stress reaction of wartime combat has been recurrently described in the military psychiatric literature at least since World War II. It is important to note that, as utilized by Solomon and others, the construct of CSR is *not* isomorphic with PTSD.

◆ CSR may be related to subsequent PTSD. In Solomon's sample, 56% of CSR soldiers had PTSD at 2 year follow-up, whereas only 18% of combat soldiers who did not have acute CSR had PTSD at 2 years.

◆ Subjects with a history of CSR had more PTSD symptoms at 2 years, even if not enough symptoms for diagnosis, than did soldiers who had no history of CSR.

◆ In PTSD cases at 1-year follow-up, intrusion symptoms were more prominent than avoidance symptoms, but not at 2 years.

◆ From a diagnostic standpoint, intrusion symptoms plus avoidance symptoms were more specific diagnostically than intrusion symptoms alone. In other words, intrusion symptoms alone appeared in subjects who were otherwise not diagnosable as having PTSD.

◆ Various factors were associated with the prevalence of PTSD. Subjects with PTSD had more readjustment difficulties (social, family, sex, employment). PTSD was associated with intrafamilial conflict, and negatively associated with family expressiveness and cohesiveness.

◆ Eighty percent of subjects with CSR who developed PTSD and 60% of cases without CSR who developed PTSD developed the PTSD soon after combat exposure.

◆ The qualitative continuity of symptoms between soldiers with CSR, soldiers without CSR but also with exposure to combat, and soldiers with PTSD (both those who had and those who did hot have CSR) was demonstrated by the fact that some symptoms were present in all four groups. Also, the relative frequencies of various symptoms within each group were similar.

◆ Delayed onset PTSD occurred in both those with acute CSR and those without CSR. In one survey of the clinical records of 150 veterans, the delayed onset rate was 10%, whereas the rate of delayed help-seeking in patients with chronic PTSD was 40%.

◆ Among soldiers with PTSD, those who had experienced previous CSR had more intense symptoms than those who had never experienced CSR.

◆ Demographic factors, including age, education, economic status, previous posttraumatic symptoms, combat exposure, and CSR, are all associated with some amount of variance in PTSD.

◆ The intensity of PTSD symptomatology declined between 2 and 3 years after combat trauma, as did general distress in soldiers with combat exposure but without PTSD, whether or not they had had CSR.

### Studies of Children

Terr (1983) documented important clinical features of PTSD in a group of children ($N = 25$) of various ages who were kidnapped and buried alive for 16 hours in a truck-trailer. When they were evaluated at 1- and 4-year follow-up, as a group the children showed an increase of the following over time: mortification or intense shame, thought suppression, denial and repression of earlier posttraumatic symptoms, unlinking of memories from affects, misperceptions, sense of foreshortened future, death dreams, and reenactment play. Most had some active fears related to the trauma, such as the fear that the kidnapper would return or that there would be another kidnapping. Terr found that all 25 children could give a fully detailed account of the traumatic events (i.e., there was little amnesia). This is different from what is found in many adults with PTSD.

Other differences from adult PTSD that were observed at the 4-year point were absence of psychic numbing and absence of intrusive dysphoric flashbacks. Also, decline in school performance was uncommon. At the 1-year follow-up of this group, classical undisguised traumatic dreams had been prominent. But in general, dreams had changed at the 4-year point to terror dreams with no recall of content, or with recall of content that was disguised with reference to the trauma.

### Studies on Former Prisoners of War

In their study of 188 ex-POWs from World War II, Kluznik and colleagues (1986) found a lifetime PTSD prevalence of 66.4% and a current prevalence of 47.3%. They reported that in this sample, aside from one possible case of delayed onset, symptoms of PTSD had begun upon repatriation and persisted, with gradual diminution over time.

In a study of 62 ex-POWs from World War II, Speed and colleagues (1989) found that 31 of 62 subjects had had PTSD during the first year after release, that the disorder had waned in 13 subjects, and that 18 still showed the disorder. In this study, there were no instances of delayed subtype. Sixteen of the 62 subjects had never had PTSD. Prewar factors did not correlate strongly with PTSD; the specific characteristics of the traumatic stressors covaried with the severity of PTSD. In almost all instances, the intensity of PTSD symptoms had declined over time, although approximately 40 years after confinement, torture, and so on, 29% still qualified for the diagnosis of PTSD.

Zeiss and Dickman (1989) reported on a questionnaire study of 442 ex-POWs from World War II (44% response rate on questionnaires sent to 1,112 persons). They found a current PTSD rate of 55.7%, with some symptoms present in 27.1%. Of the respondents, 13.8% had never been seriously troubled by PTSD symptoms, 23.5% reported being continuously troubled, and 62.2% reported being temporarily or intermittently troubled over the years. Although the data about being "troubled" are not reported as PTSD case-ness, they are mentioned here in that they are consistent (though from a group who experienced quite different traumatic stressors) with the course variability described by the Australian and Israeli studies.

Zeiss and Dickman (1989) failed to find good correlations between current symptoms and duration of, or harshness of, maltreatment during captivity. Although this finding is consistent with the results of some and inconsistent with the results of others studies on ex-POWs, I mention it here because it leads the authors to a speculation relevant to course. They speculate that trauma may not be a cumulative or additive variable, but, rather, a "critical event" or "threshold" variable such that beyond a certain critical level of trauma, increased duration or severity has little or no additional psychological impact.

The possible relevance of a concept of threshold is suggested also by such phenomena, frequently observed clinically, as 1) delayed onset; 2) the receding of chronic PTSD after many years even without formal treatment; and 3) the precipitation of PTSD many years following the initial trauma, by a stressful event (perhaps not a traumatic stressor, but rather a more ordinary stressful life event), but where the content of the symptoms refer to the earlier trauma long ago.

### National Vietnam Veterans Readjustment Study

The large National Vietnam Veterans Readjustment Study, reported in 1988 by Kulka and colleagues (1990), found a current PTSD prevalence of 15% in Vietnam veterans approximately 19 years postwar (on average), with a 30% lifetime prevalence, suggesting a slow decline of the PTSD prevalence in this population. Kulka and colleagues also found in the PTSD cases a current total comorbidity rate of approximately 50% for several other psychiatric disorders (50% total for panic disorder, general anxiety disorder, obsessive-compulsive disorder, major depression, manic episode, substance use disorder, and antisocial personality). That is, approximately 50% of Vietnam veterans with PTSD currently had at least one of these other disorders, and 50% did not. However, the *lifetime* rate of comorbidity with PTSD for the same group of disorders was 99%. The receding of the other measured disorders as indicated by these data (difference between lifetime and current prevalence rates) may bear on the longitudinal course of PTSD. Questions about this issue will be posed below.

### Buffalo Creek

Green and colleagues (1990) reported on a 12-year follow-up of 120 survivors of the 1972 flood in Buffalo Creek, West Virginia. This study found that most subjects had improved over time as measured by the Symptom Checklist—90 (SCL-90; Derogatis et al. 1973) and that the PTSD prevalence rate had changed from 44% in 1974 to 28% in 1986. Symptom severity within the PTSD groups at the two points in time had declined from a Psychiatric Evaluation Form (PEF; Endicott and Spitzer 1972) severity rating of 3.9 in 1974 to 2.7 in 1976. This study lends further support to the phenomenon of delayed PTSD. Although 61% of the total sample showed no change in PTSD diagnosis (present or absent) and 28% changed from having PTSD in 1974 to not having PTSD in 1986, 11% were not diagnosable as having PTSD in 1974 but were in 1986. The authors note, however, that any of these cases could be cyclic rather than delayed (i.e., not diagnosable in 1974, but perhaps so earlier as well as later).

## Some Key Issues

### Subthreshold PTSD (Possible DSM-IV Code: i.e., condition not attributable to a mental disorder that is a form of attention or treatment)

Regarding the occurrence of posttraumatic stress symptoms (PTSS) in persons who have insufficient symptoms to qualify for the diagnosis of PTSD, most studies reviewed here indicate that this probably occurs frequently. PTSS have long been noted in both mental health and popular literature to occur in subjects who do not show diagnosable PTSD (e.g., war veterans), particularly in the first year after exposure to traumatic stress.

The studies reviewed here indicate that PTSD, absent diagnosable PTSD, are very common not only early on, but after many years. For example, Kulka and colleagues (1990) found in Vietnam veterans that there was a current prevalence rate of 11% for having 3 to 5 symptoms of PTSD (6 are required for diagnosis) an average of 19 years after exposure to traumatic stress.

### Type of Trauma

The complexities of the relationship between type of trauma and course are indicated by the following: approximately 40 years after World War II, ex-POWs showed current PTSD prevalence rates of 50%, 47.3%, 29%, and 55.7% in four studies reviewed here, whereas the rate after 29 months among a Australian brushfire fighters was 14%. However, some of the former (ex-POWs, compounded traumas over long duration) were showing improvement in the absence of treatment, but some of the latter (fire fighters, less complex traumas over short duration) were not improving even though they were receiving treatment.

The results of this review serve as a useful reminder that the types of events producing PTSD are very different in multiple ways, including duration, complexity, content qualities, and kinds and amounts of associated losses. They also suggest that longer and more complex traumatic stress experiences may tend to produce more severe or longer-lasting PTSD (but not in everyone). The status of the literature indicates that research on the relation of type of trauma and longitudinal course is just beginning.

### Mutative Factors

With regard to factors associated with exacerbation and amelioration of PTSD over time, suggestive data are present in these studies concerning a role for coping strategies, locus of control, social support, family function, education, religion, later traumas and losses, personality, prior training or other stress inoculation factors, and various family of origin factors, including socioeconomic status and psychiatric disorder history—all in addition to nature, duration, and complexity of traumatic stress.

### Secondary Gain

None of the reports reviewed here addresses fiscal secondary gain as a significant issue. Two authors indicate that their subjects, though highly chronic, were not receiving compensation and had little interest in doing so (Archibald and Tuddenham 1965; Kluznik et al. 1986). In addition, recent data from the Department of Veterans Affairs (1989) indicate that as of 1988, only about 40,000 (4%) of approximately 900,000 Vietnam veterans who have had PTSD at some time since the war (as demonstrated by Kulka et al. 1990) have even applied for compensation for the condition. Whatever may be the relevance of fiscal secondary gain in some individual clinical cases, it appears to be considered relatively unimportant by researchers, perhaps because it is a relatively uncommon phenomenon.

### Morbidity

Some of these studies indicate that PTSD has various unfavorable impacts on adjustment and functioning over time, in that group rates are higher for employment and marital difficulties, and so on (see especially Kulka et al. 1990; Solomon et al. 1988a, 1988b). However, in most studies, a degree of disjunction can be found between presence of the disorder and level of functioning. The phenomenon of the individual who is functioning well, in the face of a significant degree of symptoms, is common. This is observed especially in the ex-POW studies referenced.

## Problems and Challenges for Research

Certain methodological problems are readily detectable in the studies reviewed and are as follows.

**Overgeneralizing.**   Most authors tend to discuss the PTSD that they are studying, although it follows a particular type of traumatic stress, as though it were *the* generic PTSD. The reports suffer from lack of qualifying language, and restraint on generalizing from, for example, PTSD in brushfire fighters after 15 hours of fire fighting, or PTSD in ex-POWs, after several years of confinement, to all PTSD from all types of traumatic stress. Greater restraint on generalizing about PTSD and a clearer focus on the limits of studies of outcomes from single trauma types are desirable.

**Measurement of stressors.**    More detailed measurement, or reporting of measurement, of the specified features of traumatic stresses encountered is needed. For example, in all of the reports by Solomon and colleagues, otherwise quite rich and valuable, there is a lack of consideration of type, duration, and qualities of the traumatic stress experienced by the combat soldiers. Variations in traumatic experiences should be considered as a variable.

As another example, McFarlane's studies are significantly constrained by limiting measurement of trauma to five factors (subject believed he/she came close to dying; says came close to panicking; sustained property damage or bereavement; and amount of time fighting fire), two of which are probably unduly subjective. Other important factors such as witnessing of deaths or seeing casualties are evidently not addressed. In contrast, the study of Kulka and colleagues (1990) casts a wider net for specific traumatic experiences and can therefore investigate the actual impact of particular features of traumatic stress more deeply.

**Caution about implying causality.**    Frequently, correlational data are presented and accompanied by language that implies causality, although the author does not directly assert it. In particular, the terms "predicts" and "explains" are used in referring to correlational variance. These terms can unscientifically lull both author and reader into thinking that causality is at hand when it may not be, and both terms should be avoided.

**Non–PTSD acute reactions.**    As the studies by Solomon and colleagues help to clarify, some PTSD clinical and research literature has tended to assume that all, or most, acute and immediate posttraumatic stress reactions or symptoms are PTSD, when in fact this is not the case. For example, many cases of acute combat stress reactions (see also Rahe 1988) represent a much more diffuse state, do not meet PTSD criteria, and do not evolve into diagnosable PTSD.

**Residual and evaporation hypotheses.**    Early in the contemporary development of PTSD as a clinical and research construct, Figley (1978) summarized two differing views in the literature reflecting 1) the stress evaporation hypothesis and 2) the residual stress hypothesis. He summarized the former view as holding that PTSS fade away over time in the absence of other psychopathology, where the latter view holds that traumatic stress per se can leave lasting effects. The studies covered in this review demonstrate that both hypotheses are consistent with available data. Some traumatic stress effects fade away with time, and some remain; the amount of fading away with time varies greatly, both from person to person, and sometimes within the same person.

**Diagnostic Interview Schedule (DIS).**    A number of population studies of PTSD have based their conclusions upon use of the Diagnostic Interview Schedule (DIS; Robins et al. 1981). McFarlane found that the DIS, when administered by a clinician, performed well at diagnosing PTSD. Kulka and colleagues (1990) also found that same effectiveness in the validation pre-test of the National Vietnam Veterans Readjustment Study, again where the instrument was administered by a clinician. However, in the large national survey by Kulka and colleagues, where the DIS-type instrument was administered by a nonclinician, it failed quite significantly, detecting only 1 in 4 of the most serious cases of PTSD. Fortunately this lack was detected through the utilization of multiple measures.

Deficiencies in the DIS or other instruments should be anticipated and countered by the use of multiple measures and any other available checks on validity, as well as by using instruments of demonstrated effectiveness in measuring PTSD. The Mississippi PTSD scale (Keane et al. 1988), a self-administered questionnaire requiring relatively little time to complete, was strongly validated in the Kulka and colleagues (1990) study and should be investigated for validity in other studies.

**Real and illusory comorbidity.**    The finding of Kulka and colleagues (1990) that the comorbidity of PTSD with a group of DIS-detected common other psychiatric disorders had declined from approximately 99% lifetime to approximately 50% currently is a striking finding concerning longitudinal course. This finding suggests multiple research hypotheses, including but not limited to the following:

1.  The DIS sorts PTSD symptoms incorrectly as other disorders when the PTSD symptoms are severe, but this effect lessens with time and decreasing PTSD symptom severity;
2.  When severe, PTSD symptoms "spread" (e.g., associated features of

anxiety or depression) and misleadingly produce other diagnoses on survey instruments such as the DIS; or

3. PTSD in early years following trauma is actually associated with other Axis I disorders that, however, fade away in some cases with time.

**Other traumatic stress outcomes.**   Clinical observation and research currently suggest that disorders in both children and adults associated with child sexual and physical abuse, such as multiple personality and borderline personality disorders, are outcomes of traumatic stress. Although these areas are not addressed as such in this review, they are noted as important topics having to do with the course of PTSD. The brief report of three cases by Goodwin (1985) illustrates how the syndrome in children following sexual abuse may be isomorphic with PTSD in adults.

# Summary of Findings on Longitudinal Course

◆ Posttraumatic stress symptoms not adding up to PTSD are quite common in response to traumatic stress, may represent a normal or healthy response to extreme or catastrophic situations, may fade in a short time, may persist as such, or may presage a case of PTSD. These should be identified in a diagnostic nomenclature as, for example, a V code in DSM-IV.

◆ There is ample evidence for acute, delayed, chronic, and intermittent or recurrent forms of PTSD, with respect to course.

◆ The correlation between length, severity, and complexity of trauma, and length, severity, and complexity of course, is partial and not absolute.

◆ Relative proportions of intrusion, avoidance, and hyperarousal symptoms in some cases probably vary over time. Recent studies indicate that on a group basis, intrusion symptoms may be more prominent in some cases initially and avoidance symptoms more prominent later; however, these data are highly preliminary.

◆ In some cases, PTSD symptoms diminish over time, probably in association with many differing factors. In other cases they do not diminish and in fact may worsen in the absence of treatment.

◆ Although acute symptoms often precede a chronic condition, delayed

PTSD may appear a significant time after traumatic stress, there having been little or no symptoms soon after the stress.
◆ Comorbidity of other psychiatric disorders with PTSD may change over time.
◆ A wide variety of factors may affect the course of PTSD, including coping mechanisms, social support, type and duration of stress, later stress, family functioning, personality, other disorders, and so on.

# References

American Psychiatric Association: Diagnostic and Statistical Manual of Mental Disorders, 3rd Edition. Washington, DC, American Psychiatric Association, 1980

American Psychiatric Association: Diagnostic and Statistical Manual of Mental Disorders, 3rd Edition, Revised. Washington, DC, American Psychiatric Association, 1987

Archibald H, Tuddenham R: Persistent stress reaction after combat: a twenty-year follow-up. Arch Gen Psychiatry 12:475–481, 1965

Department of Veterans Affairs: Post traumatic stress disorder in Vietnam veterans. Congressional Research Service Report, #89-368SPR7. Washington, DC, Library of Congress, June 1989

Derogatis LR, Lipman RS, Covi L: SCL-90: an outpatient psychiatric rating scale. Psychopharmacol Bull 9:13–28, 1973

Endicott J, Spitzer RL: What! another rating scale? The Psychiatric Evaluation Form. J Nerv Ment Dis 154:88–104, 1972

Figley CR: Stress Disorders Among Vietnam Veterans. New York, Brunner/Mazel, 1978

Goldstein G, van Kammen W, Shelly C, et al: Survivors of imprisonment in the Pacific Theater during World War II. Am J Psychiatry 144:1210–1213, 1987

Goodwin J: Post-traumatic symptoms in incest victims, in Post-Traumatic Stress Disorder in Children. Edited by Eth S, Pynoos R. Washington, DC, American Psychiatric Press, 1985, pp 157–165

Green BL, Lindy JD, Grace MC, et al: Buffalo Creek survivors in the second decade: stability of stress symptoms. Am J Orthopsychiatry 60:43–54, 1990

Keane TM, Caddell JM, Taylor KL: Mississippi Scale for combat-related posttraumatic stress disorder: three studies in reliability and validity. J Consult Clin Psychol 56:85–90, 1988

Kilpatrick DG, Saunders BE, Veronen LJ, et al: Criminal victimization: lifetime prevalence, reporting to police, and psychological impact. Crime and Delinquency 33:479–489, 1987

Kluznik J, Speed N, Van Valkenburg C, et al: 40-year follow-up of US prisoners of war. Am J Psychiatry 143:1443–1446, 1986

Kulka RA, Schlenger WE, Fairbank JA, et al: Trauma and the Vietnam War Generation. New York, Brunner/Mazel, 1990

McFarlane A: Long-term, psychiatric morbidity after a natural disaster. Med J Aust 145:561–563, 1986a

McFarlane AC: Post-traumatic morbidity of a disaster. J Nerv Ment Dis 174:4–14, 1986b

McFarlane AC: Post-traumatic phenomena in a longitudinal study of children following a natural disaster. J Am Acad Child Adolesc Psychiatry 5:764–769, 1987

McFarlane AC, Polikansky SK, Irwin C: A longitudinal study of the psychological morbidity in children due to a natural disaster. Psychol Med 17:727–738, 1987

McFarlane AC: The phenomenology of post-traumatic stress disorders following a natural disaster. J Nerv Ment Dis 176:22–29, 1988a

McFarlane AC: The longitudinal course of post-traumatic morbidity. J Nerv Ment Dis 176:30–39, 1988b

McFarlane AC: The aetiology of post-traumatic morbidity: predisposing, precipitating, and perpetuating factors. Br J Psychiatry 154:221–228, 1989

Rahe RH: Acute versus chronic psychological reactions to combat. Milit Med 153:365–373, 1988

Robins LN, Helzer JE, Cronghland JL, et al: NIMH Diagnostic Interview Schedule—Version III (PHS Publ No ADM-T-42-3 [5/8/81]). Rockville, MD, National Institute of Mental Health, 1981

Saigh PA: Anxiety, depression, and assertion across alternating intervals of stress. J Abnorm Psychol 97:338–341, 1988

Solomon Z: Combat-related PTSD among Israeli soldiers. Bull Menninger Clin 51:80–95, 1987

Solomon Z: Psychological sequelae of war: a 3-year prospective study of Israeli combat stress reaction casualties. J Nerv Ment Dis 177:342–346, 1989a

Solomon Z: A three year prospective study of post-traumatic stress disorder in Israeli combat veterans. Journal of Traumatic Stress 2:59–74, 1989b

Solomon Z, Mikulincer M: Combat stress reactions, PTSD, and social adjustment. J Nerv Ment Dis 175:277–285, 1987

Solomon Z, Mikulincer M: Psychological sequelae of war: a 2-year follow-up study of Israeli combat stress reaction casualties. J Nerv Ment Dis 176:264–269, 1988

Solomon Z, Garb R, Bleich A, et al: Reactivation of combat-related PTSD. Am J Psychiatry 144:51–55, 1987a

Solomon Z, Mikulincer M, Fried B, et al: Family characteristics and PTSD: A follow-up of Israeli combat stress reaction casualties. Fam Process 26:383–395, 1987b

Solomon Z, Weisenberg M, Schwartzwald J, et al: Post traumatic stress disorder among frontline soldiers with combat stress reaction: the 1982 Israeli experience. Am J Psychiatry 144:448–454, 1987c

Solomon Z, Benbenevisty R, Mikulincer M: A follow-up of Israeli casualties of combat stress reaction ("battle shock") in the 1982 Lebanon War. Br J Clin Psychol 27:125–135, 1988a

Solomon Z, Mikulincer M, Avitzur E: Coping, locus of control, social support and combat-related PTSD: a prospective study. J Pers Soc Psychol 55:279–285, 1988b

Solomon Z, Mikulincer M, Flum H: Negative life events, coping responses, and combat-related psychopathology: a prospective study. J Abnorm Psychol 97:302–307, 1988c

Solomon Z, Kotler M, Shaler A, et al: Delayed onset PTSD among Israeli veterans of the 1982 Lebanon War. Psychiatry 52:428–436, 1989

Speed N, Engdahl B, Schwartz J, et al: Post traumatic stress disorder as a consequence of the POW experience. J Nerv Ment Dis 177:147–153, 1989

Terr L: Chowchilla revisited: the effects of psychic trauma four years after a school-bus kidnapping. Am J Psychiatry 140:1543–1550, 1983

Zeiss R, Dickman H: PTSD 40 years later: incidence and person-situation correlates in former POWs. J Clin Psychol 45:80–87, 1989

# ◆ 2 ◆ Subtypes of Posttraumatic Stress Disorder and Duration of Symptoms

Barbara Olasov Rothbaum, Ph.D.
Edna B. Foa, Ph.D.

**Summary**     In this chapter, the authors review the course of posttraumatic stress disorder symptoms in the ensuing months after rape, criminal victimization, and other trauma to both adults and children. A high rate of spontaneous remission is noted, most of which takes place in the early months after trauma. Issues are considered for and against viewing such early, self-limited, reactions as being pathological or normal. The authors examine whether adjustment reaction eventually converts to PTSD and find there to be no such relationship.

## Statement of the Issue

Posttraumatic stress disorder (PTSD) is the only anxiety disorder for which the occurrence of an external event is specified as a diagnostic criterion. As such, it is possible to delineate its course beginning at inception. This delineation should result in consistent patterns across traumas and individuals. However, it is expected that any traumatic event, by definition, would elicit emotional distress. Therefore, it is important to distinguish between normal and pathological reactions to trauma. The initial reactions and symptomatology between normal and pathological reactions to trauma may appear similar, even in their intensity. The course would be expected, however, to deviate, with normal reactions dissipating and pathological reactions becoming chronic.

23

One important aspect that we address in this chapter is the duration of symptoms required to define a reaction to trauma as pathological (i.e., as a psychiatric disorder). On the one hand, it is important to make this distinction as early as possible in the course of the disorder to facilitate the treatment of affected individuals. On the other hand, it is important not to overdiagnose pathology and waste precious resources on individuals who are already on the road to recovery. Because the diagnosis of Adjustment Disorder in DSM-III-R (American Psychiatric Association 1987) rests in part on the duration of symptoms following a stressor, this review will also attempt to clarify the overlap between this disorder and PTSD.

Although the overall course of PTSD should be well-defined, there may be several characteristic response patterns following the trauma. Whereas some individuals become acutely distressed immediately following the incident, others may develop pathological symptoms at a later date. Accordingly, DSM-III (American Psychiatric Association 1980) distinguished two subtypes of PTSD: acute ("symptoms begin within six months of the trauma and have not lasted six months," p. 237) and chronic or delayed ("symptoms either develop more than six months after the trauma or last six months or more," p. 237). The utility of these subtypes of PTSD is addressed in this chapter.

# Methods

In our review of the literature, we gave particular attention to studies that assessed PTSD symptoms at several points starting soon following the trauma. Studies of traumatized populations that only assessed fear, anxiety, avoidance, depression, social maladjustment, impairments in self-esteem, or sexual difficulties were not included.

# Results

## Duration of Symptoms

To differentiate between duration of a normal response to trauma and a chronic pathological response, repeated assessments over time beginning soon after the trauma and assessing PTSD symptoms are necessary. Studies using such prospective methodology are summarized below.

We conducted a prospective study of rape and crime victims (E. B. Foa and B. O. Rothbaum, unpublished data, 1990) and also conducted a similar study with our colleagues (B. O. Rothbaum, E. B. Foa, and L. A. Hoge, unpublished data, 1990). Each of the following PTSD symptoms was assessed via a structured interview: reliving experiences, nightmares, flashbacks, avoidance of reminders and thoughts of the assault, impaired leisure activities, sense of detachment, blunted affect, disturbed sleep, memory and concentration difficulties, hyperalertness, increased startle response, feelings of guilt, and increased fearfulness.

Rape victims ($N = 64$) were first interviewed within 2 weeks following their assault (mean = 12.64 days) and once weekly thereafter for 12 weeks. Follow-up assessments were conducted 6 and 9 months following the assault ($N = 24$). The results indicated that at the initial interview, 94% of rape victims manifested PTSD, meeting symptomatic but not duration criteria for a diagnosis. At 1 month (mean = 35 days) postassault, 65% met criteria for PTSD. This figure decreased to 52.5% by 2 months postassault and to 47% by 3 months postassault. At 6 months postassault, 41.7% were classified as having PTSD, and at 9 months postassault, 47.1% were so classified. Thus, nearly all of the rape victims in this sample exhibited PTSD immediately following the assault, but less than half continued to meet criteria for this disorder 3 months later. The incidence of PTSD did not change appreciably after the 3-month assessment.

The results for victims of nonsexual criminal assault (simple and aggravated assault and robbery) were similar to those found for the rape victims. A majority of the crime victims responded with PTSD symptoms initially, but the incidence of PTSD decreased over time (E. B. Foa and B. O. Rothbaum, unpublished data, 1990). Approximately 1 week following assault ($N = 51$), 64.7% exhibited PTSD, decreasing to 36.7% 1 month postassault, 25% 2 months postassault, 14.6% 3 months postassault, and 11.5% 6 months following the crime ($N = 26$). At 9 months postassault, none of the 15 crime victims interviewed met criteria for PTSD. Thus, like the rape victims, most of the crime victims initially responded with PTSD symptoms that decreased substantially by 3 months postassault. Although the pattern of gradual decrease in PTSD incidence by 3 months postassault was the same for rape and crime victims, it is important to note that rape victims were more likely to develop PTSD initially and to maintain it over time.

Evidence from other populations converge with the rape and crime victims' reactions cited above to suggest that once a chronic case of PTSD has developed, it is likely to remain relatively stable over time if treatment intervention is not introduced (McFarlane 1988a, 1988b). Three hundred fifteen fire fighters were assessed for PTSD using the General Health Questionnaire (GHQ; Goldberg 1972) 4, 6, 11, and 29 months postdisaster. Sixty-nine percent of fire fighters who were symptomatic at 4 months after a fire remained such at later assessments, suggesting that PTSD at 4 months is a relatively good predictor for the chronicity of the disorder (McFarlane 1988a). Results congruent with this conclusion comes from another study with fire fighters (McFarlane 1988b). Eighty-one percent of fire fighters diagnosed as PTSD at 8 months following the fire ($N = 50$) still had PTSD at 42 months postfire. Thus, it appears that by 3–4 months posttrauma, and definitely by 6–8 months posttrauma, the course of PTSD has become chronic and can no longer be expected to subside naturally, as in a normal reaction to trauma.

Several studies attempted to assess the incidence of PTSD using a retrospective methodology. An investigation of PTSD rate in rape victims was conducted by Resnick and colleagues (H. S. Resnick, L. J. Veronen, B. E. Saunders, et al., personal communication, October 1989). Victims ($N = 33$) were interviewed 12–36 months postassault to assess the presence and duration of PTSD symptoms. The results were remarkably similar to those reported by us. Seventy-six percent (75.8%) of the rape victims reported experiencing PTSD symptoms that had been present for less than 1 month, 60.6% reported PTSD lasting at least 1 month, and 39.4% met criteria for PTSD at the time of inquiry, 12–36 months postassault.

An investigation of PTSD using a modified version of the Diagnostic Interview Schedule (DIS; Robins et al. 1981) was conducted with crime victims from a community sample of 391 adult females (Kilpatrick et al. 1987). Of those who had experienced a completed rape, 57.1% suffered from PTSD at some point following the assault, and 16.5% met PTSD criteria at the time of the inquiry (an average of approximately 15 years postassault). Of aggravated assault victims, 36.8% had PTSD at some point after the assault, and 10.5% were diagnosed as having PTSD at the time of the interview (average of 10.5 years postassault). Thus, again, a large number of victims initially responded to rape with PTSD symptoms, but a smaller number developed a chronic disorder. In addition, rape appeared to be more likely to induce PTSD than did other serious crimes not involving sexual assault.

In yet another retrospective study, lifetime and current prevalence of PTSD was investigated in a community sample of 214 adult family survivors of homicide (Kilpatrick et al. 1988). Subjects were assessed for PTSD via a 30-minute telephone interview. Twenty-nine percent of criminal homicide survivors experienced PTSD at some point, with 7.0% experiencing PTSD at the time of inquiry (which was not specified). Of the alcohol-related vehicular homicide survivors, 34.1% experienced PTSD at some point, with 2.2% experiencing PTSD at the time of inquiry. Thus, approximately one-third of homicide survivors had an occurrence of PTSD at some point following the death, but a very small percentage developed a chronic disorder.

A different picture emerged from data collected on civilians who experienced heavy shelling during wartime. Saigh (1988) assessed 12 undergraduate and graduate students at the American University of Beirut in 1983 and 1984 before and after a major offensive involving heavy shelling of the areas near the university. Structured interviews aimed at diagnosing PTSD retrospectively (approximately 1 year following the shelling) revealed that 9 of the 12 (75%) students interviewed experienced PTSD symptoms immediately following the shelling. However, the symptoms of eight of these nine spontaneously remitted within 1 month after the shelling; the remaining student developed chronic PTSD. These results are consistent with reports from World War II demonstrating that civilians during an air raid exhibited short-lived fear reactions, but very few developed intense persistent fear reactions (Rachman 1989). Findings corroborating this observation were also reported from Northern Ireland (Cairns and Wilson 1984).

Although it is not within the scope of our discussion here, it is important to note that the response of civilians following air-raid bombings differed from the response of rape victims to their trauma. A smaller percentage of the civilians developed intense persistent fear reactions in comparison to the rape and crime victims. Differences in the nature of the trauma may account for the different incidence rates. Air raids are more likely to be perceived as predictable and circumscribed, occurring only in wartime, and are not personal in nature. Rape, on the other hand, is often perceived as unpredictable, leaving its victims feeling universally vulnerable and personally violated.

There are data suggesting that the course of PTSD in children may be similar to that of adults. Children aged 5 to 13 were evaluated for PTSD approximately 1 month ($N = 159$) and 14 months ($N = 100$) following a fatal sniper attack on their school playground (Nader et al. 1990; Pynoos et al. 1987). Using the children's version of the PTSD Reaction Index (Pynoos et al. 1987) completed by an interviewer, they found that PTSD was significantly correlated with degree of exposure. At the 1-month assessment, 77% of the children who were on the playground during the attack were classified as having severe or moderately severe PTSD, and 67% of children who were in the school building had moderate PTSD. At the 14-month assessment, 74% of the children who were on the playground still manifested PTSD as compared to less than 19% of those who were in the school. The latter did not significantly differ from the unexposed group (children not at school during the attack). Thus, nearly all of the children studied who were on the playground during the attack and evidenced PTSD at the 1-month assessment were suffering from chronic PTSD at 14 months, whereas children who were less exposed to the attack (i.e., those who were inside the school) recovered sometime between 1 and 14 months postattack. A 1-month duration of symptoms was an excellent predictor of chronic PTSD in the highly exposed children, but a poor predictor for the less exposed group. Perhaps an intermediate assessment would have increased the accuracy of prediction for the entire population. The incidence rates of PTSD across different studies is summarized in Table 2–1.

McFarlane's (1988a; 1988b) data on fire fighters are not included in the table because of the manner in which these data were reported (e.g., percentage of those with PTSD at the initial assessment who remained PTSD at the subsequent assessment). Inspection of the data in Table 2–1 reveals the longitudinal course of PTSD across traumas and across studies. The similarities between the results of different investigations with similar populations supports the reliability of the findings. The rape and crime studies evidence a high incidence of PTSD initially, which decreases gradually and appears to stabilize somewhere around 3 months postassault. A certain proportion of these cases remain chronic sufferers. The civilians also respond with a high rate of PTSD initially, but almost all recover quickly. Children's reactions appear to vary with their proximity to the original trauma: most of the children in close proximity to the sniper, for example, responded with PTSD that remained chronic. However, most of the children who were not

**Table 2–1.** Incidence (%) of PTSD across studies at different times following trauma

| Study and Sample | Time Posttrauma | | | | | | | | |
|---|---|---|---|---|---|---|---|---|---|
| | 1 Week | <1 Month | 1 Month | 2 Months | 3 Months | 6 Months | 9 Months | 12–36 Months | 10–15 Years |
| Foa and Rothbaum 1990 (unpublished data) Rape | 94.0 | | 65.0 | 52.4 | 47.0 | 41.7 | 47.1 | | |
| Resnick et al. 1989 (unpublished data) Rape | | 75.8 | 60.6 | | | | | 39.4 | |
| Kilpatrick et al. 1987 Rape | | | | | | | | | 16.5 |
| Foa and Rothbaum 1990 (unpublished data) Crime | 64.7 | | 36.7 | 25.0 | 14.6 | 11.5 | 0.0 | | |
| Kilpatrick et al. 1988 Crime | | | | | | | | 10.5 | |
| Saigh 1988 Civilian | | 81.8 | 9.1 | | | | | | |
| Pynoos et al. 1987 High-exposure children | | | 77.0 | | | | 74.0 | | |
| Pynoos et al. 1987 Low-exposure children | | | 67.0 | | | | <19 | | |

in close proximity to the sniper initially responded with PTSD that tended to dissipate over time.

## Subtypes

DSM-III distinguished between two subtypes of PTSD: acute ("symptoms begin within six months of the trauma and have not lasted six months," p. 237) and chronic or delayed ("symptoms either develop more than six months after the trauma or last six months or more," p. 237). Based on clinical experience, a distinction between acute and chronic or delayed PTSD has been supported by several authors (Kolb 1983; van der Kolk 1987). Kolb (1983) noted

> That one conspicuously unique expression of Vietnam victims, the delayed stress reaction, represents only the breakdown of the conscious and unconscious psychological defense; it is seen in sudden re-emergence of panic attacks, transient explosions of rage and violence, or dissociative acting out (flashbacks). (p. 538)

Proponents of this distinction (van der Kolk and Kadish 1987) discussed psychoanalytic interpretations of delayed PTSD but offered no compelling arguments for the utility of distinguishing between delayed and acute PTSD reactions. Likewise, Kolb and Mutalipassi (1982) studied the emotional response in chronic and delayed forms of PTSD but did not report data that support the usefulness of this distinction. As suggested by McFarlane (1988a), "the definition of acute, delayed-onset, and chronic PTSDs . . . may be an arbitrary generalization based on clinical experience" (p. 34).

In the only controlled comparison available, 31 Vietnam veterans with delayed onset PTSD were compared to 32 with acute onset PTSD (Watson et al. 1988). Veterans were assessed for PTSD using a structured interview based on DSM-III criteria. No significant differences between the two groups emerged. In addition, no evidence was found to support the hypotheses that delayed onset is related to the severity of the trauma, the severity of the symptoms, repression, or previous stress history. In the above-cited studies of school children following a fatal sniper attack (Nader et al. 1990; Pynoos et al. 1987), no cases of delayed PTSD reactions were noted. That is, PTSD was present at the 14-month assessment only in those children who were diagnosed with PTSD at the 1-month assessment. Thus, it seems that the DSM-III distinction of acute, chronic, and delayed PTSD has not gained support from empirical studies. (See Chapter 1 by Blank for further review of this issue.)

## Overlapping Diagnoses

DSM-III-R specifies that symptoms should persist for 1 month before the individual can be diagnosed with PTSD. The problem has arisen regarding the diagnosis of individuals evidencing severe symptoms in the first months following a stressor but before the duration criteria for PTSD is satisfied. These individuals may require an interim diagnosis to facilitate their receiving timely treatment as well as remuneration for that treatment. Adjustment disorder has been proposed as such an interim diagnosis.

The diagnosis of adjustment disorder requires "a reaction to an identifiable psychosocial stressor (or multiple stressors) that occurs within three months of onset of the stressor(s)" (DSM-III-R, p. 330) and does not last longer than 6 months. Other diagnostic criteria include impairment in occupational and/or social functioning, or the presence of symptoms that exceed those normally expected in reaction to the stressor. This diagnosis is usually assigned when the symptoms follow a common life stress and are not severe or persistent enough to meet the diagnostic criteria for other disorders, particularly depressive or anxiety disorders. Examples of typical stressors associated with adjustment disorder listed in DSM-III-R include divorce, business or marital problems, chronic illness, leaving home, becoming a parent, and retirement.

If adjustment disorder is used as an interim diagnosis for PTSD, it follows that it should be a relatively good predictor for later development of PTSD. A longitudinal study of patients who received a diagnosis of adjustment disorder (Andreasen and Hoenk 1982) revealed differential prognoses for adults ($N = 48$) and adolescents ($N = 52$). Five years following the original diagnosis of adjustment disorder, 79% of the adults were found to be well (diagnosis free), with only 8% having experienced an intervening problem. Most of the adults who were not well at follow-up developed major depression or alcoholism but not PTSD. In adolescents, 57% were well at follow-up, with 13% having experienced an intervening problem. The adolescents' later diagnoses included schizophrenia, schizoaffective disorder, major depression, bipolar disorder, antisocial personality, alcoholism, and drug use disorder. Thus, the diagnosis of adjustment disorder appears to have represented a transient reaction in most of the adults, but was indicative of more severe problems in almost one-half of the adolescents. More importantly for the purpose of our discussion, PTSD was not observed in either group. These results suggest that adjustment disorder is not an acute form of PTSD because it did not predict its development and thus is not an appropriate interim diagnosis.

Several researchers have proposed that "Posttraumatic stress reaction" be used as a V code interim diagnosis (i.e., a condition not attributable to a mental disorder, but requiring attention or treatment). Solomon and Mikulincer (1988) described a combat stress reaction (CSR) that occurs during war (i.e., on the battlefield) and includes "restlessness, psychomotor retardation, psychological withdrawal, sympathetic activity, startle reactions, confusion, nausea, vomiting, and paranoid reactions" (Solomon and Mikulincer 1988, p. 264, from Grinker and Spiegel 1945). Solomon and Mikulincer (1988) noted: "Despite the extreme variability of this phenomenon, a common denominator can be identified: the soldier ceases to function militarily and/or begins to function in a bizarre manner that usually endangers himself and/or his comrades" (p. 264). In assessing the long-term problems of Israeli veterans from the 1982 Lebanon War, 59% of CSR cases became PTSD at 1 year postwar as compared to 16% of a veteran control group who had not manifested CSR. At 2 years postwar, 56% of CSR cases and 14% of non–CSR controls, respectively, met diagnosis for PTSD. Thus, CSR appeared to be a good predictor of later development of PTSD. Therefore, CSR or the more generic posttraumatic stress reaction, in contrast to adjustment disorder, appears to be an appropriate interim diagnosis for the period following a trauma before a diagnosis of PTSD can be assigned.

## Discussion

The studies we have discussed in this chapter indicate that the diagnosis of PTSD on the basis of symptoms 1 month after the trauma will result in overdiagnosis. This could lead to the wasting of precious resources on many who would recover without intervention. Several studies converge to indicate that the presence of PTSD at approximately 3 months posttrauma adequately predicts the chronicity of the disorder. Although the studies that suggest a 3-month posttrauma criteria included only rape and crime victims, there is no reason to assume that the 3-month criterion would not adequately apply to other types of traumas (see Table 2–1). Indeed, fire fighters' PTSD appeared to be chronic by 4 months postfire.

If a duration criterion for the diagnosis on PTSD is adopted, we will face the dilemma that, in some instances, an individual's initial reaction is so severe that a psychiatric diagnosis is warranted. As an interim diagnosis, two possibilities were discussed: adjustment disorder and posttraumatic stress reaction. Empirical evidence does not support a strong relationship between adjustment disorder and PTSD. On the other hand, the phenomenon of CSR seems to be a precursor of PTSD in most cases. However, there are very few data regarding the phenomenology of this syndrome, and all the data are derived from subjects who had been under stress during combat. The fact that 60% of CSR cases became PTSD merits intensive study of this syndrome, broadening it from a combat stress reaction to the proposed posttraumatic stress reaction.

It has also been proposed by those with extensive clinical experience with PTSD to remove the duration requirement for a diagnosis altogether. This has the advantage of acknowledging the distress following most traumas with a psychiatric diagnosis, with all the benefits accompanying a diagnosis (e.g., financial, legal, social). Removal of the duration criteria would also carry several disadvantages. The primary drawback would be the assignment of a psychiatric diagnosis, implying pathology, to individuals undergoing a normal response to trauma who will recover without intervention. These individuals may then receive unnecessary treatment and strain an already inadequate system. There is also some evidence to suggest that individuals may not profit from treatment following trauma until their condition has stabilized and become relatively chronic (Kilpatrick and Calhoun 1988).

If the duration requirement were to be eliminated, it has been suggested to label PTSD reactions within the first 3 months posttrauma as "acute," changing to "chronic" once they have persisted beyond the 3-month marker. PTSD reactions that do not arise until the 3-month point would be termed "delayed." This would eliminate the need for an interim diagnosis as well as indicate the course of the individual's PTSD. However, the previous subtypes of acute versus delayed PTSD relied on uncontrolled clinical observations, although the proposed use of these labels differs slightly from that incorporated into DSM-III-R. It is clear that some people do, in fact, have delayed PTSD, although empirical evidence reviewed here does not support the utility of this distinction. Specific recommendations for DSM-IV are provided in Appendix 2.

# References

American Psychiatric Association: Diagnostic and Statistical Manual of Mental Disorders, 3rd Edition. Washington, DC, American Psychiatric Association, 1980

American Psychiatric Association: Diagnostic and Statistical Manual of Mental Disorders, 3rd Edition, Revised. Washington, DC, American Psychiatric Association, 1987

Andreasen NC, Hoenk PR: The predictive value of adjustment disorders: a follow-up study. Am J Psychiatry 139:584–590, 1982

Cairns E, Wilson R: The impact of political violence on mild psychiatric morbidity in Northern Ireland. Br J Psychiatry 145:631–635, 1984

Goldberg DP: The Detection of Psychiatric Illness by Questionnaire. London, Oxford University Press, 1972

Grinker RR, Spiegel JP: Men Under Stress. Philadelphia, PA, Blakistan, 1945

Kilpatrick DG, Calhoun KS: Early behavioral treatment for rape trauma: efficacy or artifact? Behavior Therapy 19:421–427, 1988

Kilpatrick DG, Saunders BE, Veronen LJ, et al: Criminal victimization: lifetime prevalence, reporting to police, and psychological impact. Crime and Delinquency 33:479–489, 1987

Kilpatrick DG, Amick A, Veronen LJ, et al: Preliminary research data on post traumatic stress disorder following murders and drunk driving crashes. Paper presented at the National Organization for Victim Assistance's 14th Annual Meeting, Tucson, AZ, September 1988

Kolb LC: Return of the repressed: delayed stress reaction to war. J Am Acad Psychoanal 11:531–545, 1983

Kolb LC, Mutalipassi LR: The conditioned emotional response: a sub-class of the chronic and delayed post-traumatic stress disorder. Psychiatric Annals 12:979–987, 1982

McFarlane AC: The longitudinal course of posttraumatic morbidity: the range of outcomes and their predictors. J Nerv Ment Dis 176:30–39, 1988a

McFarlane AC: The phenomenology of posttraumatic stress disorders following a natural disaster. J Nerv Ment Dis 176:22–29, 1988b

Nader K, Pynoos R, Fairbanks L, et al: Children's PTSD reactions one year after a sniper attack on their school. Am J Psychiatry 147:1526–1530, 1990

Pynoos RS, Frederick C, Nader K, et al: Life threat and posttraumatic stress in school-age children. Arch Gen Psychiatry 44:1057–1063, 1987

Rachman S: Fear and Courage, Second Edition. New York, WH Freeman, 1989

Robins LN, Helzer JC, Croughland JL, et al: The NIMH Diagnostic Interview Schedule: its history, characteristics, and validity. Arch Gen Psychiatry 38:381–389, 1981

Saigh PA: Anxiety, depression, and assertion across alternating intervals of stress. J Abnorm Psychol 97:338–341, 1988

Solomon Z, Mikulincer M: Psychological sequelae of war: a two-year follow-up study of Israeli combat stress reaction (CSR) casualties. J Nerv Ment Dis 176:264–269, 1988

van der Kolk BA: Psychological Trauma. Washington, DC, American Psychiatric Press, 1987

van der Kolk BA, Kadish W: Amnesia, dissociation, and the return of the repressed, in Psychological Trauma. Edited by van der Kolk BA. Washington, DC, American Psychiatric Press, 1987

Watson CG, Kucala T, Manifold V, et al: Differences between posttraumatic stress disorder patients with delayed and undelayed onsets. J Nerv Ment Dis 176:568–572, 1988

# ◆ 3 ◆ What Constitutes a Stressor? The "Criterion A" Issue

John S. March, M.D., M.P.H.

***Summary*** In deciding whether or not an event is traumatic, several factors need to be considered; these include the importance of stressor intensity and duration, and whether physical injury, loss, death, or exposure to the grotesque took place. The relation between PTSD symptoms and stressor magnitude or unusualness is described. Subjective response to the event is considered, including perceived life threat, potential for physical violence, fear, and helplessness. Finally, the author reviews conceptual issues and breadth of definition and suggests a definition for a traumatic stress.

## Introduction

Posttraumatic stress disorder (PTSD), the most recent of many names for the syndrome resulting from exposure to life-threatening stressors (Trimble 1985), remains a controversial addition to the psychiatric diagnostic inventory. While there is little dispute over the face validity of the diagnosis among clinicians, there is considerable uncertainty among researchers about the scope of the diagnosis, particularly as it pertains to understanding potentially traumatic interactions between persons and environmental events. Nowhere is this debate more apparent than in the literature addressing the PTSD stressor (A) criterion.

## Statement of the Issue

PTSD never occurs de novo but always requires an initiating event, usually assumed to be "catastrophic" in its quantitative and qualitative aspects, viz. its "intensity" and "nature." By specifying that such events 1) should evoke "significant symptoms of distress in most people" and 2) be "outside the range of usual human experience," DSM-III (American Psychiatric Association 1980, pp. 236–238) implicitly included subjective perception as well as environmental objectivity within the PTSD construct. Despite the implicit requirements for threat appraisal, however, DSM-III overtly followed Axis IV when describing qualifying events, requiring that the related concepts of severity and unusualness be "based on the clinician's assessment of the stress an 'average' person in similar circumstances and with similar sociocultural values would experience" (pp. 236–238).

Although DSM-III-R (American Psychiatric Association 1987) continued the approach initiated with DSM-III, several important modifications were made to the stressor criteria (Brett et al. 1988). First, in an effort to refine the phenomenological criteria to better reflect anxiety-related symptoms, DSM-III-R notes that stressors in PTSD are "usually experienced with intense fear, terror, and helplessness" (p. 247). Second, in addition to direct experience of the stressor, DSM-III-R provides for PTSD following visual (witnessing an event) and verbal (hearing about an event) mediation. Finally, DSM-III-R provides examples of qualifying events within the criteria set as well as nonqualifying events within the accompanying text, separating these events along quantitative and qualitative dimensions. Thus DSM-III-R also acknowledges (without operationalizing) the importance of subjective perception while continuing to frame PTSD as a stressor-driven anxiety disorder.

In anticipation of DSM-IV, arguments have been presented for reformulating the stressor criterion in favor of subjective perception as contrasted to tightly defined objective characteristics. Advocates of the former position suggest that the stressor criterion be abolished altogether or defined as an event shocking the individual (Solomon and Canino 1990); advocates of the latter suggest that the stressor criterion be reformulated in terms of generic features common to environmental events shaping PTSD phenomenology. In this chapter, I review the empirical evidence on these and related issues in an effort toward furthering a revised definition of traumatic stress (i.e., Criterion A in the diagnosis of PTSD as provided in DSM-III-R).

Specific questions addressed include the following:

◆ Do stressors demonstrate a quantitative (dose-response) effect?
◆ Do specific stressor characteristics predispose to PTSD or are stressors

equipotent with response varying as a function of intensity?

◆ What is the evidence for subjective perception (i.e., the appraisal of threat) in the generation of PTSD?

◆ Does the stressor criterion need to be specifically modified for children?

◆ How might incorporating both objective and subjective perspectives affect the operating characteristics of the stressor criterion or the criteria set as a whole?

# Method

As part of a larger work on the nosology of PTSD (March 1990), the psychiatric and psychological literature was systematically searched for empirical studies relating to traumatic stress.

In the absence of a unifying theory for PTSD, both terminology and underlying theoretical constructs must be clearly defined in order to maximize information content and to delineate generalizability. In this chapter, stress is defined as an organismic response to the experience of an external event or stimulus. Such an event is termed a stressor in the presence of a related psychiatric disorder. With respect to theoretical bias, my discussion in this chapter is informed by an empirical multicausal/multieffect or interactionist premise in which PTSD is viewed as a stressor-driven anxiety disorder. (See the Epilogue for further comments in interactions between event and vulnerability.)

# Review of the Literature

Abundant historical and clinical experience links life-threatening events with the development of PTSD or PTSD-like symptoms (Ettedgui and Bridges 1985). A brief examination of typical PTSD-inducing events (Table 3–1) reveals that virtually all are capable of eliciting extreme fear and the perception of absolute helplessness. Most are events external to the affected individual; one, a sudden illness, is a life-threatening internal event that is generally perceived as being outside individual control. All involve the potential for physical injury or death and exhibit the capacity to elicit affectively laden visual imagery.

The events listed in Table 3–1 uniformly demonstrate face validity within the overall PTSD construct. Thus it is not surprising to find that PTSD re-

Table 3–1.    Characteristic PTSD stressors

| | |
|---|---|
| Combat | Natural disasters |
| Criminal assault | Human disasters |
| Rape | Witnessing homicide |
| Accidental injury | Witnessing sexual assault |
| Industrial accident | Sudden illness (example: |
| Automobile accident | acute myocardial |
| Hostage | infarction) |
| Prisoner of war (POW) | Severe burns |

searchers have focused almost without exception on these or comparable stimuli as demonstrated in Tables 3–2 (design features) and 3–3 (findings), which summarize the 40 articles meeting the search criteria described earlier. With four exceptions, selected articles utilize DSM-III or DSM-III-R criteria. Most are either case series, case-control, or correlational in design. Only five studies examine the issue of comorbidity, an important methodological deficit. In addition, variations in theoretical interpretation and the use of diverse instruments for operationalizing both dependent and independent variables render the comparisons reported below of uncertain validity.

## Quantitative Aspects

The dominant conclusion to be drawn from these studies is that stressor magnitude is directly proportional to the subsequent risk of developing PTSD. Sixteen of 19 studies examining the question of stressor intensity endorse a dose-response relationship. Furthermore, this finding occurs within and across a variety of settings—natural disaster, combat, prisoner of war (POW) experiences, criminal victimization, and accidents—and transcends methodological approach as well, implying that it is quite robust. No study identifies a threshold effect, although one suggests that a threshold phenomenon may operate with respect to mediating variables (Shore et al. 1986), a finding mirrored in research endeavors: the more transactional approaches, embodied in appraisal models, are focused on daily hassles (Lazarus 1984). PTSD, occurring in the context of high-intensity events, is the subject of the least transactional models.

Nevertheless, despite general agreement that increasing intensity (dose)

**Table 3–2.**　Design features of studies relating stressor to symptoms

| Reference | ST | N | DX | Set | Design | Comorbid |
|---|---|---|---|---|---|---|
| Burstein 1985 | MXD | 73 | CDSM3 | O/I | CS | – |
| Shore et al. 1986 | DIS | 1025 | SDSM3 | COM | EPI | + |
| Friedman et al. 1986 | COMB | 58 | SDSM3 | OVA | COR | – |
| Solomon et al. 1988a | COMB | 104 | SDSM3 | OSC | COR | – |
| Miller et al. 1988 | POW | 62 | CDSM3R | OVA | CS | – |
| Snow et al. 1988 | COMB | 2858 | SDSM3 | COMM | EPI | – |
| Zeiss and Dickman 1989 | POW | 442 | SDSM3 | COMM | EPI | – |
| Speed et al. 1989 | POW | 62 | SDSM3 | OVA | CS | – |
| Woolfork and Grady 1988 | COMB | 48 | SDSM3 | OSC | CC | – |
| Pitman et al. 1987 | COMB | 33 | SDSM3R | OVA | CC | – |
| Laufer et al. 1985 | COMB | 251 | PDSM3 | COMM | EPI | – |
| Green et al. 1985a | NDIS | 117 | PDSM3 | OSC | COR | – |
| Green et al. 1989 | COMB | 200 | SDSM3 | OSC | COR | + |
| Horowitz et al. 1980 | MXD | 66 | PDSM3 | OSC | CS | – |
| Solomon and Flum 1988 | COMB | 716 | SDSM3 | OSC | CC | – |
| Green et al. 1983 | MDIS | 117 | PDSM3 | OSC | COR | – |
| Foy and Card 1987 | COMB | 297 | SDSM3 | COMM | EPI | – |
| Kilpatrick et al. 1989 | CRIME | 391 | SDSM3 | COMM | EPI/CC | – |
| Amick et al. 1989 | CRIME | 1166 | SDSM3 | COMM | EPI | – |
| Mikulincer and Solomon 1988 | COMB | 262 | SDSM3 | OSC | COR | – |
| Solomon et al. 1988b | COMB | 255 | SDSM3 | OSC | COR | – |
| Pitman et al. 1989 | COMB | 156 | SDSM3 | COMM | CS | – |
| Madakasira and O'Brien 1987 | NDIS | 116 | DSM3 | COMM | CC | – |
| Green and Berlin 1987 | COMB | 61 | DSM3 | I/OVA | COR | – |
| Foy et al. 1987 | COMB | 43 | DSM3 | IVA | CC | – |
| Frye and Stockton 1982 | COMB | 88 | DSM3 | COMM | COR | – |
| Pearce et al. 1985 | COMB | 90 | DSM3 | I/OC | CC | – |
| Breslau and Davis 1987 | COMB | 69 | SDSM3 | IVA | CC | + |
| Saigh 1989 | COMB | 840 | SDSM3 | COMM | CC | – |
| Kilpatrick et al. 1987 | CRIME | 391 | SDSM3 | COMM | EPI | – |
| McFarlane 1988 | MXD | 4 | CDSM3 | OC | CS | – |
| Helzer et al. 1987 | MXD | 2493 | SDSM3 | COMM | EPI | + |
| Penk et al. 1981 | COMB | 208 | PDSM3 | IVA | CC | – |

Table 3–2.   Design features of studies relating stressor to symptoms (continued)

| Reference | ST | N | DX | Set | Design | Comorbid |
|-----------|-----|-----|-------|------|--------|----------|
| McLeer et al. 1988 | CSA | 31 | SDSM3 | OC | CS | – |
| Solomon et al. 1987 | COMB | 716 | SDSM3 | OSC | CS | – |
| Pynoos et al. 1987 | CRIME | 159 | SDSM3 | COMM | EPI | – |
| Kiser et al. 1988 | CSA | 10 | CDSM3 | OC | CS | – |
| Stoddard et al. 1989 | BURN | 16 | CDSM3 | I | CS | + |

*Note.* ST = stressor, *N* = number, DX = diagnosis, Set = setting, Design = study design, Comorbid = comorbidity; MXD = mixed, NDIS = natural disaster, COMB = combat, POW = prisoner of war, MDIS = man-made disaster, CRIME = criminal victimization, CSA = childhood sexual abuse, MI = myocardial infarction, BURN = burned; CDSM3 = clinical DSM-III, SDSM3 = structured DSM-III, PDSM3 = pre-DSM-III, SDSM3R = structured DSM-III-R; O = outpatient, I = inpatient, SC = specialty clinic, VA = veterans administration, COMM = community; CS = case series, EPI = epidemiologic, COR = correlational, CC = case-control; + = controlled, – = uncontrolled.

of exposure is proportional to PTSD risk, it can be argued that discriminating quantitatively between "catastrophic" and "everyday" events presents an impossible conundrum. What is "outside the range of usual experience" for one person may be extraordinary for another. Certain experiences that are prominently associated with PTSD (i.e., rape and childhood sexual abuse) are unfortunately too prevalent to be considered unusual, despite the fact that such stressors encompass the "generic" stressor dimensions described below. Furthermore, it is difficult to imagine how chronic exposure to low-level threat can be quantitatively reconciled with more severe events of shorter duration. As has been pointed out, long-term exposure may have different effects than single-trial learning in any case (Kiser et al. 1988).

To determine whether stressors of lower magnitude (nonqualifying under DSM-III-R) exhibit the capacity to induce PTSD, the stressor/event must be framed as the dependent variable, an approach taken in 3 of the 40 studies. Burstein (1985) found that 8 of 73 patients in an outpatient clinical series met the phenomenological criteria for PTSD without meeting DSM-III-R criteria for stressor severity. Nonqualifying stressors included marital disruption, children's illegal activities, collapse of adoption arrangement, and death of a loved one.

In the St. Louis subset of the Epidemiologic Catchment Area (ECA) study, Helzer and colleagues (1987) found that miscarriage, a spouse's affair, and poisoning were associated with PTSD, although less commonly than were rape or Vietnam War combat exposure. Solomon and Canino (1990)

**Table 3–3.**    Findings from studies relating stressors to symptoms

| Reference | ST | Quant | Qual | Comments |
|---|---|---|---|---|
| Burstein 1985 | COMB | ne | ne | 8/73 met B, but not Acriterion /IES scores are comparable |
| Shore et al. 1986 | NDIS | dr | + | bereavement contributes to anxiety more than depression |
| Friedman et al. 1986 | COMB | dr | ne | |
| Solomon et al. 1988a | COMB | dr | + | foul-ups – / CSR + / summed experience important |
| Miller et al. 1988 | POW | dr | ne | Japanese > German exposure / Japanese > German symptoms |
| Snow et al. 1988 | COMB | dr | ne | PTSD varies with interpretation of stressor / diffuse stress + |
| Zeiss and Dickman 1989 | POW | – | + | higher rank reduces risk / Japanese = German POW risk |
| Speed et al. 1989 | POW | dr | + | injury, torture, mental status change, weight loss, witnessing, relocation, recalling suffering + |
| Woolfolk and Grady 1988 | COMB | dr | ne | |
| Pitman et al. 1987 | COMB | ne | + | scripts of actual trauma most potent |
| Laufer et al. 1985 | COMB | dr | + | abusive violence, race + |
| Green et al. 1985a | MDIS | dr | + | bereavement, life threat, perceived threat + / witnessing + / philos coping – / denial, interpersonal coping + |
| Green et al. 1989 | COMB | dr | + | special assignments + / exposure to grotesque death + / loss, injury – |
| Horowitz et al. 1980 | MXD | ne | + | IES scores = between accidents, object loss |
| Solomon and Flum 1988 | COMB | ne | + | |
| Green et al. 1983 | MDIS | ne | + | family, rescue > fire group / bereav, subj distress + |
| Foy and Card 1987 | COMB | dr | ne | |
| Kilpatrick et al. 1989 | CRIME | dr | + | life threat, injury, rape + |
| Amick et al. 1989 | CRIME | dr | + | indirect victimization + / crim = vehicular homicide |
| Mikulincer and Solomon 1988 | COMB | ne | + | "controllability" + |
| Solomon et al. 1988b | COMB | ne | + | emotional, distancing, coping + |
| Pitman et al. 1989 | COMB | ne | + | problem-focused coping – / wounding + |
| Madakasira and O'Brien 1987 | COMB | – | – | injury, property damage – |
| Green and Berlin 1987 | COMB | dr | ne | |

**Table 3–3.** Findings from studies relating stressors to symptoms (continued)

| Reference | ST | Quant | Qual | Comments |
|---|---|---|---|---|
| Foy et al. 1987 | COMB | dr | ne | wounds, kill civilian, third tour in Vietnam + |
| Frye and Stockton 1982 | COMB | dr | + | wounding – / extensive locus of control + / positive attitude at entry + |
| Pearce et al. 1985 | COMB | ne | ne | war trauma > noncombat |
| Breslau and Davis 1987 | COMB | dr | + | atrocities + / buddy killed + / separated from unit + |
| Saigh 1989 | COMB | dr | + | witnessing, hearing about + in children |
| Kilpatrick et al. 1987 | CRIME | ne | ne | high prevalence: rape > assault > burglary / low reporting of rape |
| McFarlane 1988 | MXD | ne | ne | PTSD in blind patients |
| Helzer et al. 1987 | MXD | ne | + | males: wounded in combat, seeing someone die / females: physical attack / few lower magnitude + |
| Penk et al. 1981 | COMB | dr | ne | heavy > light combat + |
| McLeer et al. 1988 | CSA | ne | + | father > stranger > trusted adult, older child < younger adult |
| Solomon et al. 1987 | COMB | ne | + | CSR without PTSD lowest in symptoms |
| Pynoos et al. 1987 | CRIME | dr | ne | exposure to sniper + |
| Kiser et al. 1988 | CSA | ne | + | chronic sexual abuse + |
| Stoddard et al. 1989 | BURN | + | ne | high lifetime, low point prevalence / parent's symptoms predicted child's |

*Note.* ST = stressor, Quant = quantitative variable, Qual = qualitative variables including stressor dimensions and subjective perception; MXD = mixed, NDIS = natural disaster, COMB = combat, POW = prisoner of war, MDIS = man-made disaster, CRIME = criminal victimization, CSA = childhood sexual abuse, MI = myocardial infarction, BURN = burned; ne = not examined, dr = dose-response, the = threshold response; under "Quant" and "Qual" + = present, – = absent; under "Comments" + means contributes, – means does not contribute to PTSD risk, CSR = combat stress reaction, IES = Impact of Event Scale.

found that PTSD symptoms, particularly reexperiencing symptoms, were more prevalent in persons experiencing common events (money problems, household illness/injury) than in persons exposed to a natural disaster. Finally, Burstein (1985) and Horowitz and colleagues (1980) both found little difference in scores between groups meeting and not meeting the PTSD stressor criterion on the Impact of Event Scale (IES; Horowitz et al. 1979), suggesting that differences between "catastrophic" and "everyday" stressors might not be as great as DSM-III-R implies.

It is important to note, however, that the methods of operationalizing the theoretical construct in these studies might have failed to adequately capture the fear-conditioning inherent in the disorder. Moreover, the IES is not a satisfactory substitute for diagnosing PTSD. Recent evidence in the life event literature suggests that stressors may indeed confer limited phenomenologic specificity, with object loss associated with depressive symptoms and threat with symptoms of anxiety (Finley-Jones and Brown 1981). Unfortunately, there are no data in the life events literature on the crucial question of whether lower magnitude stressors reliably induce the phenomenology of PTSD in contrast to other psychiatric outcomes.

## Qualitative Dimensions

What composes stressor magnitude? Most studies, especially those correlating summed stressor indices and PTSD symptomatology, contribute little to answering this question in empirical terms. Proposed "generic" characteristics include magnitude, rate of change, duration, unpredictability, lack of preparedness, and lack of prior experience, but an adequate typology is not yet available (Green et al. 1985b). Nevertheless, assuming that it is possible to disentangle stressor characteristics from related dimensions of intensity and subjective impact, the PTSD literature lends limited support to several event-specific dimensions found within and across stressor types.

Of the 24 studies reporting qualitative effects, injury was positively correlated to PTSD in 5 studies (Foy et al. 1987; Helzer et al. 1987; Kilpatrick et al. 1989; Pitman et al. 1989; Speed et al. 1989) and unrelated in 3 (Foy and Card 1987; Frye and Stockton 1982; Green et al. 1989); bereavement was positive in 4 (Breslau and Davis 1987; Green et al. 1983, 1985a; Shore et al. 1986) and unrelated in 1 (Green et al. 1989); participating in or witnessing combat-related atrocities was positive in 4 studies (Breslau and Davis 1987; Foy et al. 1987; Laufer et al. 1985; Speed et al. 1989) and exposure to grotesque death in 2 others (Green et al. 1983; Helzer et al. 1987); witnessing death was positive in 4 studies (Green et al. 1983, 1985a; Saigh 1989; Speed et al. 1989) and hearing about death in another 3 (Amick et al. 1989; Green et al. 1983; Saigh 1989). Rape (Helzer et al. 1987; Kilpatrick et al. 1987, 1989), torture (Speed et al. 1989), property damage (Shore et al. 1986), and life threat (Kilpatrick et al. 1987) were also independent risk factors in some studies.

In addition, PTSD following the murder of civilians during wartime (Foy et al. 1987) and acting as the agent of criminal homicide (Harry and Resnick 1986) stimulates questions about the necessity of being the object of threat and about the subjective importance of role. In any case, the dimensions of threat to life, severe physical harm or injury, exposure to grotesque death, and loss and/or injury of a loved one are at least modestly correlated to the likelihood of developing PTSD (also see Green 1990 for a discussion of stressor dimensions). Furthermore, although "diffuse" stress can be associated with PTSD (Foy et al. 1987; Snow et al. 1988; Solomon et al. 1988a), it is likely that increasing prevalence of these constituent elements is proportional to an increased risk of intensity as well as to the shape of subsequent symptom pattern. Consistent with this perspective, Pearce and associates (1985) found that combat is a more potent inducer of PTSD symptomatology than noncombat stressors.

## Subjective Perception

Echoing the quantitative and qualitative descriptors of PTSD-inducing events, the most salient empirically documented aspects of subjective perception involve the perception of life threat, perceived potential for physical violence, the experience of extreme fear, and the attribution of personal helplessness. Implicit in this picture is the assumption that the impact of the event on the individual determines whether or not the event is traumatic (i.e., whether an event becomes a stressor). This is a crucial distinction because, even under horrendous circumstances, most individuals do not develop PTSD (March 1990). Clinical evidence suggests that relatively low objective magnitude may rarely induce PTSD, given sufficient vulnerability in the exposed individual.

Unfortunately, there is relatively little inferential and even less empirical support for this position in the empirical PTSD literature. In part, this reflects constraints imposed by the objective slant of the stressor criterion in DSM-III-R. More important, perhaps, is the fact that attributional style is best studied prospectively, a difficult objective to implement with the events listed in Table 3–1.

Nevertheless, given the caveat that the data are highly confounded and largely unreplicated, inferential evidence of subjectivity includes findings that higher rank is protective (Zeiss and Dickman 1989). Other findings include that rape is a more potent variable than associated crime-related factors such as injury (Kilpatrick et al. 1989), that "foul-ups" are negatively correlated with PTSD in Israeli combat veterans (Solomon et al. 1988a), that a positive attitude toward service entry is a risk factor for Vietnam combat-related PTSD (Frye and Stockton 1982), that sexual abuse by fathers exceeds that by strangers in potency, and that sexual abuse by another older child is much less potent a risk factor (McLeer et al. 1988), and that stressor-specific scripts are more potent than generic scripts in inducing psychophysiologic responses in persons with PTSD (Pitman et al. 1987).

More direct evidence for the importance of subjective perception is provided by studies demonstrating that higher levels of perceived threat (Green et al. 1985b), perception of suffering (Speed et al. 1989), cognitive perception of low controllability (Frye and Stockton 1982; Mikulincer and Solomon 1988), and coping styles dominated by emotional responses or by denial (Green et al. 1985b; Solomon et al. 1988b) exacerbate the risk for or course of PTSD. These lines of research are post hoc, however, and are thus subject to undetectable ascertainment, motivation set, and response set biases.

## The Stressor in Children

The need to incorporate an element of subjective perception within the stressor criterion is perhaps more apparent with regard to children than adults. Children exposed to severe stressors clearly develop PTSD (Eth and Pynoos 1985). Furthermore, exposed children demonstrate a symptom profile similar to that seen in adults (Lyons 1987). Just as the features of the disorder vary with the developmental stage of the child (Terr 1985), however, the variety of environmental events capable of producing PTSD phenomenology also varies in children from that seen in adults (Gislason and Call 1982). Children, as illustrated by the fact that parental symptoms reliably predict a child's PTSD symptoms (Stoddard et al. 1989), are less readily conceptualized as distinct from their environmental surroundings (Emde 1989). Thus, reactive attachment disorder, seen in very young children exposed to grossly pathogenic parenting, is correctly conceptualized in DSM-III-R as an interpersonal problem rather than as a posttraumatic stress disorder. Comparable issues obtain with respect to chronic sexual abuse, physical abuse, and severe emotional neglect in children from dysfunctional families. The status of PTSD in children has been reviewed by Eth (in press) and by McNally (see Chapter 4).

# Discussion

The usual format for evaluating PTSD is to use exposure to the stressful event as the entry criterion or independent variable. For the most part, clinical decisions in this regard are dichotomous. One is either exposed or not and the stressor is validated by the presence or absence of the phenomenological criteria. Although this used to be the case for research studies as well, the current practice is to operationalize exposure by utilizing event-specific indices, thereby requiring a cutoff score below which persons do not meet criteria for the disorder. Using an operationalized measure of combat severity, Snow and colleagues (1988) demonstrate that varying the A criteria results in substantial variation in the percentage of veterans meeting criteria for the diagnosis. Narrowly defining exposure restricted the diagnosis to 1.8% of the population; a much broader definition permitted a maximum diagnostic rate of 15%, essentially the percentage of individuals meeting the phenomenological criteria.

Whether conceived dimensionally or dichotomously, all attempts to arbitrarily limit the stressor criteria will necessarily result in a certain percentage of false negative and/or positive diagnoses. In principle, the effects of modifying the criterion along a quantitative axis can be measured (Hsaio et al. 1989). On the other hand, it is difficult to predict what impact the introduction of subjective factors might have on the operating characteristics of the criteria set. In this context, it may be heuristically useful to consider the implications of adopting a broad versus a narrow formulation of the stressor criterion.

At its extreme, a broad view would in essence abolish the stressor criterion through teleologically defining the stressor by its results. The quantitative or "catastrophic" threshold for the diagnosis would be eliminated with preference given to a purely subjective interpretation. Any stressor capable of inducing PTSD phenomenology would qualify. In practical terms, the elimination of a quantitative threshold would potentially open the diagnostic category to every individual with intrusive recollections of a distressing event, however mild. Stated differently, because reexperiencing demonstrates virtually 100% sensitivity, it would serve as a de facto entry criterion, given that a stressor would necessarily have to be reexperienced in order to be traumatic. Theoretically, this would present a problem only if the C and D criteria lack sufficient specificity to prevent false positive diagnoses. Practically, however, the application of the C and D criteria is far from uniform, primarily because PTSD is not uniformly viewed as a stressor-driven anxiety disorder (March 1990). Unless the diagnostic criteria are applied uniformly, however, the resultant increase in diagnostic heterogeneity would soon swamp both research and clinical endeavors. The forensic and social policy repercussions of this result could in themselves be catastrophic. On the positive side, broadening the stressor criteria would foster essential research designed to ascertain which qualitative and quantitative factors are in fact associated with PTSD phenomenology in which persons subject to which events.

What of the narrow view? At its narrowest, advocates of this position might favor excluding subjective perception, restricting the diagnosis of PTSD to individuals who have experienced events such as those most commonly associated with PTSD in the research and historical literatures. Consistent with clinical experience and the data of Snow and colleagues (1988), this position would minimize the false-positive rate by limiting entry into the diagnostic process. The principal advantage of this approach is its ability to minimize diagnostic heterogeneity, a key element is establishing diagnostic reliability and predictive validity. On the other hand, a narrow formulation of the stressor criterion would increase false negative diagnoses by eliminating those persons who, presumably because of heightened vulnerability, develop PTSD after experiencing events of relatively low magnitude. Clinically, this may represent a substantial number of individuals, given that the prevalence of lower magnitude events is likely to be greater (with the possible exception of sexual assault) than that of high-magnitude events. Similarly, the reliance on a highly restrictive (essentially dichotomous) stressor criterion would eliminate from consideration as research subjects a pool of individuals rich in information content.

In summary, both the narrow and broad formulations of the stressor criterion pose problems in that they invite theoretical confusion, lack clinical utility, and fail to optimize the operating characteristics of criteria set. Moreover, they fail to represent the empirically derived multicausal/multieffect approach that will be required to better understand potentially traumatic interactions between people and environmental events.

# Conclusion

The empirical literature is clear that stressor dose—determined in part by life threat, physical injury, object loss, and perhaps grotesquery—is the major risk factor for the development of PTSD. Two principal issues vis-à-vis reformulating the stressor criterion remain: 1) How should subjective perception be reconciled with objective descriptors? and 2) What about PTSD risk from lower magnitude events? The empirical information necessary to decide these issues is unavailable. Neither is it currently possible to predict how changes in the stressor criterion might affect the operating characteristics of the criteria set as a whole, especially since other criterion variables may also change in DSM-IV.

Although one argument for mandating subjective perception was to qualify individuals making high-magnitude attributions to low-magnitude events and thus to qualify those events as well, this approach unnecessarily blurs the distinction between event magnitude and subjective perception. Moreover, including subjective perception in the criterion itself raises the impossible conundrum of timing. Most individuals will make helplessness attributions during or immediately after a potentially traumatic event; some will not, however. In this context, helplessness attributions are consistent clinically with symptom development, not necessarily with the event itself. Thus, absent additional information, subjective perception will necessarily remain where it currently resides, namely in the realm of vulnerability assessment.

Similarly, persons symptomatic after lower magnitude events will continue to fall in the transitional and dimensional gray area that characterizes our psychiatric taxonomy. This said, a two-part stressor criterion incorporating both objective and subjective features could be considered. An example of such a definition is given in Table 3–4. The objective features are reasonably well supported in the empirical literature; the subjective features reflect the perceptual correlates of typical PTSD-inducing events. Consideration should be given to empirically testing these recommendations.

---

**Table 3–4.**   Proposed stressor criteria

---

1) The person has experienced, witnessed, or been confronted with an event (or events) involving an actual or threatened encounter with violent death or physical injury.

2) The person's response involved intense fear, personal helplessness, and/or horror.

# References

American Psychiatric Association: Diagnostic and Statistical Manual of Mental Disorders, 3rd Edition. Washington, DC, American Psychiatric Association, 1980

American Psychiatric Association: Diagnostic and Statistical Manual of Mental Disorders, 3rd Edition, Revised. Washington, DC, American Psychiatric Association, 1987

Amick A, Kilpatrick D, Resnick H, et al: Public health implications of homicide for surviving family members. Paper presented at the Society for Behavioral Medicine, San Francisco, CA, April 1989

Breslau N, Davis G: Posttraumatic stress disorder: the etiologic specificity of wartime stressors. Am J Psychiatry 144:578–583, 1987

Brett E, Spitzer R, Williams J: DSM-III-R criteria for posttraumatic stress disorder. Am J Psychiatry 145:1232–1236, 1988

Burstein A: Posttraumatic stress disorder. J Clin Psychiatry 46:554, 1985

Emde R: The infant's relationship experience: developmental and affective aspects, in Relationship Disturbances in Early Childhood. Edited by Sameroff A, Emde R. New York, Basic Books, 1989

Eth S: Post-traumatic stress disorder in childhood, in Handbook of Child and Adult Psychopathology. Edited by Herzen M, Last C. New York, Pergamon (in press)

Eth S, Pynoos R: Posttraumatic Stress Disorder in Children. Washington, DC, American Psychiatric Press, 1985

Ettedgui E, Bridges M: Posttraumatic stress disorder. Psychiatr Clin North Am 8:89–103, 1985

Finley-Jones R, Brown G: Types of stressful live events and the onset of anxiety and depressive disorders. Psychol Med 11:803–815, 1981

Foy D, Card J: Combat-related posttraumatic stress disorder etiology: replicated findings in a national sample of Vietnam-era men. J Clin Psychol 43:28–31, 1987

Foy D, Sipprelle R, Rueger D, et al: Etiology of posttraumatic stress disorder in Vietnam veterans: analysis of premilitary, military and combat exposure influences. J Consult Clin Psychol 43:643–649, 1987

Friedman M, Schneiderman C, West A: Measurement of combat exposure, posttraumatic stress disorder, and life stress among Vietnam combat veterans. Am J Psychiatry 143:537–539, 1986

Frye S, Stockton R: Discriminant analysis of posttraumatic stress disorder among a group of Vietnam veterans. Am J Psychiatry 139:52–56, 1982

Gislason I, Call J: Dog bite in infancy. J Am Acad Child Psychiatry 21:203–207, 1982

Green B: Defining trauma: terminology and generic stressor dimensions. Journal of Applied Social Psychology 20:1632–1642, 1990

Green B, Grace M, Lindy J, et al: Levels of functional impairment following a civilian disaster: the Beverly Hills Supper Club fire. J Consult Clin Psychol 51:573–580, 1983

Green B, Grace M, Gleser G: Identifying survivors at risk, long-term impairment following the Beverly Hills Supper Club fire. J Consult Clin Psychol 53:672–678, 1985a

Green B, Lin de J, Grace M: Posttraumatic stress disorder: toward DSM IV. J Nerv Ment Dis 173:406–411, 1985b

Green B, Lindy J, Grace M, et al: Multiple diagnosis in posttraumatic stress disorder. J Nerv Ment Dis 177:329–335, 1989

Green M, Berlin M: Five psychosocial variables related to the existence of post-traumatic stress disorder symptoms. J Clin Psychol 43:643–49, 1987

Harry B, Resnick P: Posttraumatic stress disorder in murderers. J Forensic Sci 3:609–613, 1986

Helzer J, Robins L, McEvoy L: PTSD in the general population. N Engl J Med 317:1630–1634, 1987

Horowitz M, Wilner N, Alvarez W: Impact of Event Scale: a measure of subjective stress. Psychosom Med 41:209–218, 1979

Horowitz M, Wilner N, Kaltreider N, et al: Signs and symptoms of posttraumatic stress disorder. Arch Gen Psychiatry 37:85–92, 1980

Hsiao J, Bartko J, Polter W: Diagnosing diagnoses: receiver operating characteristic methods and psychiatry. Arch Gen Psychiatry 46:664–667, 1989

Kilpatrick D, Saunders B, Veronen L, et al: Criminal victimization: lifetime prevalence, reporting to police, and psychological impact. Crime and Delinquency 33:479–489, 1987

Kilpatrick D, Saunders B, Amick-McMullan A, et al: Victim and crime factors associated with the development of post-traumatic stress disorder. Behavior Therapy 20:199–214, 1989

Kiser L, Ackerman B, Brown E, et al: Post-traumatic stress disorder in young children: a reaction to purported sexual abuse. J Am Acad Child Adolesc Psychiatry 27:645–649, 1988

Laufer R, Brett E, Gallops M: Dimensions of posttraumatic stress disorder among Vietnam veterans. J Nerv Ment Dis 173:538–545, 1985

Lazarus R: Puzzles in the study of daily hassles. J Behav Med 4:375–389, 1984

Lyons J: Posttraumatic stress disorder in children and adolescents. Developmental and Behavioral Pediatrics 8:349–356, 1987

Madakasira S, O'Brien K: Acute posttraumatic stress disorder in victims of a natural disaster. J Nerv Ment Dis 175:286–290, 1987

March J: The nosology of post-traumatic stress disorder. Journal of Anxiety Disorders 4:61–82, 1990

McLeer S, Deblinger E, Atkins M, et al: Post-traumatic stress disorder in sexually abused children. J Am Acad Child Adolesc Psychiatry 33:650–654, 1988

McFarlane A: Posttraumatic stress disorder and blindness. Comp Psychiatry 29:558–560, 1988

Mikulincer M, Solomon Z: Attributional style and combat-related posttraumatic stress disorder. J Abnorm Psychol 97:308–313, 1988

Miller T, Martin W, Spiro K: Traumatic stress disorder: diagnostic and clinical issues in former prisoners of war. Compr Psychiatry 30:139–148, 1988

Pearce K, Schauer A, Garfield N, et al: A study of post traumatic stress disorder in Vietnam veterans. J Clin Psychol 44:9–14, 1985

Penk W, Robinowitz R, Roberts W, et al: Adjustment differences among male substance abusers who vary in degree of combat experience in Vietnam. J Consult Clin Psychol 49:426–437, 1981

Pitman R, Orr S, Forgue D, et al: Psychophysiologic assessment of posttraumatic stress disorder imagery in Vietnam combat veterans. Arch Gen Psychiatry 44:970–975, 1987

Pitman R, Altman B, Macklin M: Prevalence of posttraumatic stress disorder in wounded Vietnam veterans. Am J Psychiatry 146:667–669, 1989

Pynoos R, Frederick C, Nader K, et al: Life threat and posttraumatic stress in school-age children. Arch Gen Psychiatry 44:1057–1063, 1987

Saigh P: The development of posttraumatic stress disorder pursuant to different modes of traumatization. Paper presented at the 97th annual convention of the American Psychological Association, New Orleans, LA, August 1989

Shore J, Tatem E, Vollmer W: Evaluation of mental effects of disaster: Mount St. Helen's eruption. Am J Public Health 76:76–83, 1986

Snow B, Stellman J, Stellman S, et al: Post-traumatic stress disorder among American Legionnaires in relation to combat experience in Vietnam. Environ Res 47:175–195, 1988

Solomon S, Canino G: Appropriateness of the DSM-III-R criteria for post-traumatic stress disorder. Compr Psychiatry 31:227–237, 1990

Solomon Z, Flum H: Life events, combat stress reactions, and PTSD. Soc Sci Med 26:319–325, 1988

Solomon Z, Weisenberg M, Schwarzwald D, et al: Posttraumatic stress disorder among front-line soldiers with a combat stress reaction: the 1982 Israeli experience. Am J Psychiatry 144:448–454, 1987

Solomon Z, Benbenevisty R, Mikulincer M: A follow-up of Israeli casualties of combat stress reaction ('battle shock') in the 1982 Lebanon war. Br J Clin Psychol 27:125–135, 1988a

Solomon Z, Mikulincer M, Flum H: Negative life events, coping responses, and combat-related psychopathology: a prospective study. J Abnorm Psychol 97:302–307, 1988b

Speed N, Engdahl B, Schwartz J, et al: Posttraumatic stress disorder as a consequence of the POW experience. J Nerv Ment Dis 177:147–153, 1989

Stoddard F, Norman D, Murphy J. A diagnostic outcome study of children and adolescents with severe burns. J Trauma 29:471–477, 1989

Terr L: Psychic trauma in children and adolescents. Psychiatry Clin North Am 8:815–835, 1985

Trimble M: Posttraumatic stress disorders: history of a concept, in Trauma and Its Wake. Edited by Figley CR. New York, Brunner/Mazel, 1985, pp 5–14

Woolfolk R, Grady D: Combat-related PTSD. J Nerv Ment Dis 176:107–111, 1988

Zeiss R, Dickman H: PTSD 40 years later: incidence and person-situation correlates in former POWs. J Clin Psychol 45:80–87, 1989

◆

# Section II:

# Clinical Phenomenology: Symptomatic Manifestations in Different Patients

◆

# ◆ 4 ◆ Stressors That Produce Posttraumatic Stress Disorder in Children

### Richard J. McNally, Ph.D.

**Summary**     The author reviewed studies of childhood posttraumatic stress disorder (PTSD) on the basis of stressor (natural disaster, warfare, violent crime, severe burns, sexual abuse, accidents). PTSD was common after warfare, criminal violence, burns and serious accidents but was less consistent after sexual abuse. Most of the clinical symptoms were observed in traumatized children, although uncertainty surrounds the frequency of some symptoms.

## Statement of the Issue

Most research on PTSD as based on criteria in DSM-III (American Psychiatric Association 1980) or DSM-III-R (American Psychiatric Association 1987) concerns adults rather than children. Only recently have psychopathologists systematically studied the effects of traumatic stressors on children (Eth and Pynoos 1985; Lyons 1987; McNally 1991; Pynoos 1990; Sugar 1989; Terr 1985).

## Method

Articles in the literature on childhood PTSD were identified systematically; identified papers varied greatly in methodological quality, as befitting a relatively new research area such as childhood PTSD. Early studies usually involved either unstructured interviews with children or questionnaires that assessed symptoms but did not provide psychiatric diagnoses. Some researchers used DSM-III in unstructured interviews or applied these criteria in chart review studies. Thirteen studies involved

**Table 4–1.** Studies involving structured interviews and either DSM-III or DSM-III-R criteria

| Stressor Type | Reference |
| --- | --- |
| Mother's sexual assault witnessed | Pynoos and Nader 1988 |
| Fatal school shooting | Schwarz and Kowalski 1991 |
| Sniper attack | Pynoos et al. 1987 |
| Concentration camp | Kinzie et al. 1986 |
| Warfare | Arroyo and Eth 1985 |
| | Saigh 1989 |
| Severe burns | Stoddard et al. 1989 |
| Sexual abuse | Kiser et al. 1988 |
| | McLeer et al. 1988 |
| Sexual abuse or physical abuse | Livingston 1987 |
| Sexual abuse/incest | Sansonnet-Hayden et al. 1987 |
| Flood | Earls et al. 1988 |
| Boating accident | Martini et al. 1990 |

structured interviews and either DSM-III or DSM-III-R criteria (Table 4–1).

The text of this chapter addresses only those studies involving either DSM-III or DSM-III-R criteria (see Table 4–2 regarding stressor types and these criteria). Pre-DSM-III studies, however, occasionally provided considerable detail on posttraumatic signs and symptoms. Accordingly, data from these reports are summarized in Tables 4–3, 4–4, and 4–5.

# Results

Childhood PTSD studies are organized by stressor type (natural disasters, warfare, violent crime, severe burns, sexual abuse, and accidents).

## Natural Disasters

Most disaster research has involved either anecdotal or questionnaire data (Blom 1986; Burke et al. 1982; Dollinger 1985; Dollinger et al. 1984; Galante and Foa 1986; Gislason and Call 1982; McFarlane 1987, 1988; Milne 1977; Newman 1976). In two studies, however, researchers applied DSM-III criteria. Handford and colleagues (1986) interviewed 35 children and their parents 18 months after the Three Mile Island nuclear accident. Families were randomly sampled from those living within 30 miles of the accident. The children ranged in age from 6 to 19 years (mean age = 13.2 years). Although there were no cases of PTSD, four children received a DSM-III diagnosis: "anxiety disorder" (2), dysthymic disorder (1), and conduct disorder (1). As noted by the authors, this incidence is consistent with that found in the general population (Gould et al. 1981). Although 24 of these families had to evacuate the area temporarily, no one was hurt, and no homes were damaged. Accordingly, this incidence constituted more of a threat of disaster than a disaster per se.

Earls and colleagues interviewed 39 children and their parents 1 year after a severe flood ravaged their rural Missouri community (Earls et al. 1988). The researchers used the child and parent versions of the Diagnostic Interview for Children and Adolescents (DICA, DICA-P; Welner et al. 1987) to interview the children and parents separately. No child had DSM-III PTSD, although some children experienced PTSD symptoms. Three children (10%), each with a preexisting disorder, met criteria for DSM-III ad-

**Table 4–2.** Stressor types and either DSM-III or DSM-III-R in children

| Stressor Type | # of Ptsd Cases (%) | Reference |
|---|---|---|
| Parental homicide witnessed | 16 (100) | Malmquist 1986 |
| Mother's sexual assault witnessed | 10 (100) | Pynoos and Nader 1988 |
| Sexual abuse | 9 (90) | Kiser et al. 1988 |
| Sniper attack | 27 (77) | Pynoos et al. 1987 |
| Boating accident | 3 (60) | Martini et al. 1990 |
| Concentration camp | 19 (48) | Kinzie et al. 1986 |
| Sexual abuse | 14 (48) | McLeer et al. 1988 |
| Exposure to war | 10 (33) | Arroyo and Eth 1985 |
| Child snatching | 6 (33) | Terr 1983b |
| Severe burns | 9 (30) | Stoddard et al. 1989 |
| School shooting | 17 (27) | Schwarz and Kowalski 1991 |
| Exposure to war | 230 (27) | Saigh 1991 |
| Sexual abuse | 0 (0) | Sansonnet-Hayden et al. 1987 |
| Incest | 0 (0) | Sirles et al. 1989 |
| Parental violent death | 0 (0) | Payton and Krocker-Tuskan 1988 |
| Flood | 0 (0) | Earls et al. 1988 |
| Incest | 0 (0) | Krener 1985 |
| Sexual/physical abuse | 0 (0) | Livingston 1987 |
| Three Mile Island | 0 (0) | Handford et al. 1986 |

justment disorder with depressed mood. There were no differences in prevalence of symptoms or diagnoses as a function of sex or age. The degree of exposure to the flood was unrelated to the number of symptoms.

**Summary.**    Two natural disaster studies involved assessment for DSM-III PTSD (Earls et al. 1988; Handford et al. 1986). Neither reported any cases of PTSD, although adjustment disorders and some PTSD symptoms were noted. Other disaster studies have involved standardized questionnaires, but in no study was the full range of DSM-III symptoms assessed (e.g.,

---

**Table 4–3.**    Percentage of children exhibiting DSM-III-R reexperiencing symptoms

---

**Recurrent and intrusive distressing recollections of the event (in young children, repetitive play in which themes or aspects of the trauma are expressed)**

| | |
|---|---|
| 100 | Witness to parental homicide |
| 97 | Sniper attack |
| 90 | Witness to mother's sexual assault |
| 88 | Fatal school shooting |
| 72 | Kidnapping [posttraumatic play] |
| 13 | Brushfire [posttraumatic play] |

**Recurrent distressing dreams of the event**

| | |
|---|---|
| 100 | Witness to parental homicide |
| 100 | Kidnapping |
| 80 | Witness to mother's sexual assault |
| 63 | Sniper attack |
| 55 | Concentration camp |
| 30 | Fatal school shooting |
| 25 | Flood |
| 13 | Brushfire |

**Suddenly acting or feeling as if the traumatic event were recurring (includes a sense of reliving the experience, illusions, hallucinations, and dissociated [flashback] episodes, even those that occur upon awakening or when intoxicated)**

| | |
|---|---|
| 100 | Witness to parental homicide [flashbacks] |
| 73 | Sex ring abuse |
| 70 | Sexual abuse |
| 39 | Fatal school shooting |
| 25 | Flood |
| 13 | Kidnapping [hallucinations] |
| 0 | Kidnapping [flashbacks] |

**Intense psychological distress at exposure to events that symbolize or resemble an aspect of the traumatic event, including anniversaries of the trauma**

| | |
|---|---|
| 100 | Kidnapping |
| 90 | Sexual abuse |
| 70 | Witness to mother's sexual assault |
| 56 | Witness to parental homicide |
| 25 | Fatal school shooting |

McFarlane 1987). In summary, there is little evidence that disasters routinely produce PTSD in children. It is possible, however, that specific events that can occur during a natural disaster may trigger PTSD (e.g., witnessing the death of a family member).

## Warfare

Until recently, investigators have not directly assessed the effects of war on children (Ziv and Israeli 1973). For example, assessment of British

---

**Table 4–4.**   Percentage of children exhibiting DSM-III-R avoidance symptoms

**Efforts to avoid thoughts or feelings associated with the trauma**
| | |
|---|---|
| 94 | Sniper attack |
| 80 | Witness to mother's sexual assault |
| 75 | Witness to parental homicide |
| 72 | Kidnapping |
| 58 | Concentration camp |
| 23 | Fatal school shooting |

**Efforts to avoid activities or situations that arouse recollections of the trauma**
| | |
|---|---|
| 90 | Sexual abuse |
| 89 | Sniper attack |
| 80 | Witness to mother's sexual assault |
| 69 | Witness to parental homicide |
| 52 | Fatal school shooting |

**Inability to recall an important aspect of the trauma (psychogenic amnesia)**
| | |
|---|---|
| 0 | Kidnapping |
| 0 | Witness to parental homicide |

**Markedly diminished interest in significant activities (in young children, loss of recently acquired developmental skills such as toilet training or language skills)**
| | |
|---|---|
| 90 | Witness to mother's sexual assault |
| 66 | Sniper attack |
| 48 | Concentration camp |
| 41 | Fatal school shooting |

**Feeling of detachment or estrangement from others**
| | |
|---|---|
| 80 | Witness to mother's sexual assault |
| 59 | Sniper attack |
| 39 | Fatal school shooting |

**Restricted range of affect (e.g., unable to have loving feelings)**
| | |
|---|---|
| 50 | Witness to parental homicide |
| 48 | Fatal school shooting |

**Sense of a foreshortened future (e.g., does not expect to have a career, marriage, or children, or a long life)**
| | |
|---|---|
| 92 | Kidnapping |
| 14 | Fatal school shooting [expects not to live to age 70] |
| 0 | Sexual abuse |

children exposed to aerial bombing during World War II involved interviews with their parents; the children themselves were rarely interviewed. Those studies have been reviewed by Terr (1985).

Three studies have employed DSM-III criteria in the assessment of war-related PTSD in children. Arroyo and Eth (1985) interviewed 30 Central American refugees, aged 17 years or younger, who were referred for psychiatric evaluation. Twenty-eight subjects were from El Salvador; the others were from Nicaragua. All were exposed to war-related trauma before their arrival in the United States. Two teenaged subjects were combatants who had participated in the torture and killing of their fellow citizens. Following a full psychiatric evaluation, Arroyo and Eth diagnosed DSM-III PTSD in 10 children (33%) and adjustment disorder in 9 others (30%).

Kinzie and colleagues (1986) conducted standardized psychiatric interviews with 40 high school students who had been imprisoned between ages

**Table 4–5.**    Percentage of children exhibiting DSM-III-R arousal symptoms

**Difficulty falling or staying asleep**

| | |
|---|---|
| 88 | Witness to parental homicide |
| 77 | Sniper attack |
| 70 | Witness to mother's sexual assault |
| 40 | Concentration camp |
| 30 | Fatal school shooting |

**Irritability or outbursts of anger**

| | |
|---|---|
| 14 | Fatal school shooting |

**Difficulty concentrating**

| | |
|---|---|
| 70 | Witness to mother's sexual assault |
| 66 | Sniper attack |
| 55 | Concentration camp |
| 33 | Fatal school shooting |

**Hypervigilance**

| | |
|---|---|
| 100 | Kidnapping |
| 100 | Witness to mother's sexual assault |

**Exaggerated startle response**

| | |
|---|---|
| 91 | Sniper attack |
| 80 | Witness to mother's sexual assault |
| 67 | Fatal school shooting |
| 50 | Concentration camp |

**Physiologic reactivity upon exposure to events that symbolize or resemble an aspect of the traumatic event (e.g., a woman who was raped in an elevator breaks out in a sweat when entering any elevator)**

| | |
|---|---|
| 39 | Kidnapping |
| 23 | Fatal school shooting |

8 and 12 in Cambodian concentration camps between 1975 and 1979. After 2 years of living in refugee camps, they emigrated to the United States at approximately age 14. The children had witnessed many deaths, had endured forced labor, beatings, and starvation, and had experienced separation from their families. The interviews were conducted 4 years after the children had left Cambodia.

The 40 students (25 boys) ranged in age from 14 to 20 (mean age = 17). Twenty students (50%) had DSM-III PTSD; 5 (12%), 1 (2%), and 15 (38%) had Research Diagnostic Criteria (RDC) major, minor, and intermittent depressive disorder, respectively. Three (8%) had DSM-III panic disorder, and 7 (18%) had DSM-III generalized anxiety disorder (GAD).

Among the 20 PTSD cases, 17 (85%) had a concurrent depressive disorder. There were no instances of schizophrenia, antisocial conduct, and drug or alcohol abuse. Interrater reliability for the PTSD diagnosis was 85%.

The investigators also interviewed six students who had fled Cambodia before Pol Pot secured power. These control subjects reported few symptoms and were assigned no diagnoses. Hence emigration alone was insufficient to account for the psychopathology found in the traumatized students.

Classroom data indicated that traumatized students were withdrawn, but not disruptive (Sack et al. 1986). Despite their emotional problems, the traumatized students did not differ from the control children in terms of academic performance.

Kinzie and associates (1986) found no relationship between psychiatric status and age, sex, or the type of trauma experienced (e.g., death of a family member). However, 13 of the 14 students (93%) living alone or with foster parents received a diagnosis, whereas only 12 of 26 students (46%) living with a nuclear family member received a diagnosis. The researchers suggested that the reestablishment of contact with family members mitigated trauma-related symptoms.

At 3-year follow-up, Kinzie and associates (1989) used structured interviews to establish DSM-III-R PTSD in 48% of the 30 subjects studied. Applying DSM-III-R criteria to the original data, the authors noted that three subjects who had been diagnosed as DSM-III PTSD cases failed to meet DSM-III-R criteria, whereas two others would have been diagnosed as PTSD cases had DSM-III-R PTSD criteria been available. Thus, 48% of the subjects originally met DSM-III-R PTSD criteria.

Saigh (P. A. Saigh, personal communication, October 1989) interviewed 840 Lebanese children, ranging in age from 9 to 12 years old, who had been referred for psychological evaluation because of emotional problems related to their exposure to war. According to their responses, 273 (32%) met DSM-III PTSD criteria. Two counseling psychologists then evaluated the taped and written transcripts of the Inventory administration and jointly diagnosed 230 (27%) of the children as PTSD cases. Of these 230 cases, 58 (25%), 128 (56%), 13 (6%), and 31 (14%) had been traumatized either through direct experience, observation, verbal mediation, or some combination thereof.

**Summary.**   Three studies have involved the structured assessment of DSM-III PTSD in children exposed to war-related trauma (Arroyo and Eth 1985; Kinzie et al. 1986; Saigh 1991). In contrast to early reports of minimal distress in children exposed to warfare (e.g., World War II air raids), these recent studies have uncovered rates of PTSD ranging from 27% to 48%.

## Violent Crime

Researchers have studied the responses of children exposed to kidnapping, sniper fire, or the rape or murder of a parent. Child abuse, including sexual molestation, will be covered in a subsequent section.

In six studies, either DSM-III or DSM-III-R criteria were used. Terr (1983b) evaluated 18 children who had been either abortively or successfully kidnapped by the parent with whom they were not living. Six (33%) children met DSM-III criteria for PTSD, whereas five others (28%) exhibited the "aftereffects of severe fright" (p. 151). The PTSD cases ranged in age from 2 to 7 at the time of the childsnatching and were evaluated soon thereafter. Detailed descriptions of symptoms were not provided, but nightmares and posttraumatic play were noted.

Malmquist (1986) interviewed 16 children, ranging in age from 5 to 10, who had witnessed the murder of one of their parents. All children met DSM-III criteria for PTSD. The children were anxious, restless, hypervigilant, and exhibited impaired concentration and memory. Most exhibited declines in school performance (94%). The children expressed anger over the event, but not overt guilt. They experienced no amnesia for the event; details were recalled vividly. Indeed, unpredictable recollections were termed "flashbacks" by Malmquist. Among 50% of the children, acting-out behavior such as thievery and vandalism developed after the event. No child became psychotic.

Payton and Krocker-Tuskan (1988) reviewed the medical records of 21 children who had lost a parent through homicide ($n = 18$) or violent suicide ($n = 3$). Four had witnessed their parent's death. The children were referred by social service agencies and schools for psychiatric evaluation of a variety of behavior problems. Most were evaluated between the ages of 5 and 9 and had experienced parental loss before the age of 5 (71%). Nine received comprehensive psychological, social, and psychiatric evaluations. Of these 9, the following DSM-III diagnoses were assigned: overanxious disorder ($n = 4$), dysthymic disorder ($n = 2$), conduct disorder ($n = 2$), and adjustment disorder ($n = 1$). There were no cases of PTSD. The authors note the difficulty in ascribing the children's behavioral problems to the traumatic event of violently losing a parent. Most of these children came from impoverished, violent neighborhoods and had witnessed numerous acts of violence.

Pynoos and Nader (1988) interviewed 10 children ranging in age from 5 to 17 years old who had been referred for psychiatric evaluation after having witnessed the sexual assault of their mothers. All children met DSM-III criteria for PTSD. The investigators also used the Post-Traumatic Stress Disorder (PTSD) Reaction Index (Pynoos et al. 1987) to quantify the severity of PTSD symptoms. Nine children scored in the severe range, and one child scored in the moderate range of severity. A -.51 correlation between Index scores and age indicated that as age increased, symptoms decreased. Symptoms noted included constricted affect and hypervigilance in school-age and adolescent subjects, and posttraumatic play involving simulated sexual activity in five school-age children.

Pynoos and colleagues (1987) studied 159 children, ranging in age from 5 to 13 years old, who were exposed to a sniper attack on an elementary school playground in Los Angeles. They obtained systematic reports of PTSD symptoms by using the PTSD Reaction Index scale. Sex, age, and ethnicity did not influence symptoms, but proximity to the sniper did. Children who were closest to the sniper had more severe PTSD than did those who were less in danger. Of those children on the playground during the attack, 77% had moderate to severe levels of PTSD.

Schwarz and Kowalski (1991) studied 64 children, ranging in age from 5 to 14 years old, who experienced varying degrees of exposure to a fatal shooting at an elementary school in the affluent Chicago suburb of Winnetka. The revised PTSD Reaction Index was administered via interview 8 to 14 months after the shooting. Although questions about hypervigilance and amnesia were inadvertently omitted from the interview, 27% of children met DSM-III-R criteria for PTSD. Asking a series of questions relevant to the symptom of foreshortened future, Schwarz and Kowalski found that 15% reported they would live to be less than 70, 19% would not have children, 13% would not get married, and 2% see the future as all bad.

**Summary.**   Six studies have involved the application of DSM-III or DSM-III-R criteria to children exposed to violent crime (Malmquist 1986; Payton and Krocker-Tuskan 1988; Pynoos and Nader 1988; Pynoos et al. 1987; Schwarz and Kowalski 1991; Terr 1983b). With one exception (Payton and Krocker-Tuskan 1988), these studies indicate that exposure to criminal violence produce rates of PTSD ranging from 27% to 100%.

## Severe Burns

Stoddard and colleagues (1989) used structured interviews (DICA-C, DICA-P) to establish DSM-III diagnoses in 30 children and adolescents, aged 7 to 19, who had been severely burned. Approximately half of the children had been burned at age 2 or younger. A control group of 30 children attending a health maintenance organization (HMO) clinic were also interviewed. Interrater reliability for the DICA-C was 92%. Of the burn patients, 30% met lifetime criteria for PTSD, whereas 6.7% currently had PTSD. Overanxious disorder was present in 30% (33% lifetime), phobias in 47% (both current and lifetime), enuresis in 10% (33% lifetime), and major depression in 3% (27% lifetime). That many of the patients were burned before the age of 2 may account for the low prevalence of PTSD.

**Summary.**   Only one study has involved the formal assessment of PTSD in patients with a serious medically related trauma (Stoddard et al. 1989), although Nir (1985) claimed that PTSD occurred in childhood cancer patients "almost without exception" (p. 131). However, he provided no data to substantiate this statement.

## Sexual Abuse

The effects of sexual abuse on children have been controversial. Indeed, some authors question whether it constitutes a trauma (for a review, see Browne and Finkelhor 1986). In any event, researchers have studied the topic in several ways. First, some investigators have studied the long-term effects of childhood sexual abuse by determining its prevalence in the histories of adult psychiatric patients (Beck and van der Kolk 1987; Bryer et al. 1987; Herman et al. 1989). Unfortunately, it cannot be concluded that abuse caused the disorder. Moreover, such subjects are a biased sample; abused children who suffer no persistent ill effects will not be subjects in such studies.

Second, investigators have studied adults who had been sexually abused as children. For example, Lindberg and Distad (1985) described 17 female outpatients, ranging in age from 24 to 44, who had experienced incest in childhood. All met DSM-III criteria for PTSD. Again, the time lag between childhood trauma and adulthood psychiatric disorder makes it difficult to infer causality.

Third, investigators have studied child victims via interview or questionnaires without assigning psychiatric diagnoses (Burgess et al. 1984, 1987; Einbender and Friedrich 1989; Goldston et al. 1989; Gomes-Schwartz et al. 1985). Based on such methods, Browne and Finkelhor (1986) estimated that between 46% to 66% of sexually abused children exhibit significant psychological impairment. Although these studies document that sexual abuse harms children in many cases, they do not reveal whether the *syndrome* of DSM-III-R PTSD is a common outcome.

In six studies, however, psychiatric diagnoses were assigned to sexually abused children. After reviewing the charts of 22 young female incest victims, Krener (1985) found that 15 received a DSM-III diagnosis. Adjustment disorder with mixed emotional features was the modal diagnosis. She noted, however, that "several" probably had PTSD.

Using the DICA, Livingston (1987) assessed 13 sexually abused children (mean age = 9.7 years) and 15 physically abused children (mean age = 10 years); all were psychiatric inpatients. Among the sexually abused children, the most common diagnoses were major depression with psychotic features (77%), attention deficit disorder (69%), overanxious disorder (62%), separation anxiety (54%), and oppositional disorder (62%). Among the physically abused children, the most common diagnoses were conduct disorder (87%), attention deficit disorder (73%), and oppositional disorder (53%). There were no cases of PTSD in either group.

Kiser and colleagues (1988) evaluated 10 children, aged 2 to 6 years, who were apparent victims of sexual abuse at a day-care center. The children were interviewed and treated approximately 4 to 6 months after the alleged abuse. Based on self-report, parent report, and clinical observation, therapists assigned DSM-III-R PTSD diagnoses to 9 children. Unlike older children described by Terr (1983a), these children did not exhibit a sense of foreshortened future or omen formation.

McLeer and associates (1988) used structured interviews (DICA and DICA-P) and standardized questionnaires to determine the frequency of PTSD in 31 sexually abused children. The children were assessed an average of 8 months following the last occurrence of abuse. They ranged in age from 3 to 16 years with a mean age of 8.4 years. DSM-III-R PTSD was diagnosed in 48% of the sample—75% of those abused by their natural father, 67% of those abused by strangers, 25% of those abused by trusted adults, and in none of those abused by an older child. Many children who did not meet PTSD criteria nevertheless experienced PTSD symptoms. One or more re-experiencing symptoms were exhibited by 81% of the children in the study, three or more avoidant behaviors were exhibited by 48%, and symptoms of autonomic hyperarousal were exhibited by 64%. Moreover, 58% scored 12 or higher on the Children's Depression Inventory (Kovacs 1985), thereby suggesting they had clinical depression.

Sansonnet-Hayden and colleagues (1987) used the Diagnostic Interview for Children (DISC; A. J. Costello, C. S. Edelbrock, M. K. Dulcan, R. Kalas, and S. H. Klaric, unpublished data, June 1984) to assess 54 consecutive admissions to an inpatient adolescent psychiatric unit. Of these subjects, 17 reported a history of either intra- or extrafamilial sexual abuse (38% of girls, 24% of boys). Within the abused group, the principal DSM-III diagnoses were major depression ($n = 10$), conduct disorder ($n = 4$), oppositional disorder ($n = 1$), and dual diagnosis of major depression and conduct disorder ($n = 2$). Depression was common in the nonabused group (57%). There were no cases of PTSD.

In the largest study to date, Sirles and colleagues (1989) interviewed 207 victims of intrafamilial child sexual abuse who presented to an outpatient child psychiatry clinic. Only 38% had an Axis I diagnosis. The most frequent conditions were adjustment disorders (usually with depressed mood; 28%), conduct disorder (5%), and disorders with physical manifestations (3%). There were no cases of PTSD. The closer the relationship of the offender to the child, the older the child, the longer the duration of abuse, the occurrence of additional physical abuse, the greater the frequency of abuse, and a history of alcohol abuse in the offender were all significantly associated with the presence of an Axis I syndrome in the victim.

**Summary.**  Six studies have involved the application of DSM-III or DSM-III-R criteria to cases of child sexual abuse (Kiser et al. 1988; Krener 1985; Livingston 1987; McLeer et al. 1988; Sansonnet-Hayden et al. 1987; Sirles et al. 1989). Four of these reported no cases of PTSD, whereas the other two reported rates of 48% and 90%. Clearly, there is no uniform outcome associated with child sexual abuse.

## Accidents

Martini and colleagues (1990) used the revised version of the PTSD Reaction Index to evaluate five children who were injured when a speedboat crashed into spectators watching the Pittsburgh Regatta. The researchers also used this instrument to interview the parents about their traumatized children. Three of the children met DSM-III-R criteria for PTSD as confirmed by either self-report or parental report.

**Summary.**  Recent reports suggest that serious accidents (e.g., capsized ship; Yule and Williams 1990) produce PTSD symptoms in children, but in only one published study did investigators apply structured interviews enabling either DSM-III or DSM-III-R diagnoses (Martini et al. 1990).

## Discussion

Rates of PTSD vary widely across stressor types (Table 4–2). PTSD seems most closely associated with events that are sudden and unexpected rather than predictable or expected (e.g., witnessing the sexual assault of one's mother versus incest), involve trauma of human design (e.g., concentration camp versus flood), and involve a close brush with death (e.g., sniper attack). Indeed, some stressors (e.g., sexual abuse) are associated with a diversity of outcomes and not solely with classic PTSD.

Few research studies provide complete information on specific PTSD symptoms, although the frequency with which certain symptoms occur can be gleaned from some reports (Tables 4–3, 4–4, and 4–5). As apparent from Tables 4–3 through 4–5, there are unanswered questions concerning symptom profiles in childhood PTSD. For example, to what extent do children experience flashbacks, psychogenic amnesia, and foreshortened future? In three studies, flashbacks were explicitly addressed. In one study, 100% of the cases experienced flashbacks (Malmquist 1986), whereas in another, none did (Terr 1979). In the third study, flashbacks were mentioned, but no percentage was given (Burgess et al. 1984). Schwarz and Kowalski (1991) noted that 39% of children exposed to a fatal school shooting reported suddenly feeling that the event was recurring, thereby suggesting the presence of flashbacks.

Amnesia was addressed in only two studies (Malmquist 1986; Terr 1979); no instances were found in either investigation. A sense of a foreshortened future was noted in 92% of the subjects in one study (Terr 1983a), and in none of the cases in a second study (Kiser et al. 1988). Although Schwarz and Kowalski (1991) did not ask about foreshortened future as such, they did note that 14% of their subjects did not expect to reach the age of 70. Irritability or outbursts of anger are often reported, but it is generally unclear whether irritability preceded or resulted from the trauma. In only one study did researchers document that increases in irritability occurred following the trauma (Schwarz and Kowalski 1991). Finally, when researchers do not note particular symptoms, it is unclear whether they failed to probe for them or whether subjects did not experience them.

## Conclusions

Although "subtraumatic" events may produce PTSD in some individuals (Spitzer and Williams 1985), the research literature indicates that exposure to violence (e.g., crime, warfare) triggers PTSD in children more consistently than do other putatively traumatic stressors (e.g., natural disasters). Therefore, it is unlikely that broadening the stressor criterion will enable the identification of hitherto undetected cases of PTSD, at least in children. It is possible, of course, that further research using DSM-III-R criteria and structured interviews will reveal higher rates of PTSD than those reported in the extant literature.

Research indicates that sexual abuse does not routinely produce PTSD in children. Indeed, it is questionable whether this stressor is uniquely associated with any particular psychopathological syndrome. Disasters also do not routinely produce the disorder in children.

In summary, there is no compelling reason for altering the DSM-III-R criteria to accommodate the presentation of the disorder in children. *However,* there is a paucity of controlled, empirical research concerning certain symptoms (e.g., sense of a foreshortened future, amnesia, flashbacks, irritability). It is unclear whether researchers assessed for these symptoms, failed to find them, and therefore do not discuss them, or whether they simply did not assess for them. Additional research involving structured interviews with children and parents is needed to determine the frequency with which these symptoms occur. Such research would illuminate and perhaps strengthen the case for different presentations of the disorder in children and adults.

# References

American Psychiatric Association: Diagnostic and Statistical Manual of Mental Disorders, 3rd Edition. Washington, DC, American Psychiatric Association, 1980

American Psychiatric Association: Diagnostic and Statistical Manual of Mental Disorders, 3rd Edition, Revised. Washington, DC, American Psychiatric Association, 1987

Arroyo W, Eth S: Children traumatized by Central American warfare, in Post-Traumatic Stress Disorder in Children. Edited by Eth S, Pynoos RS. Washington, DC, American Psychiatric Press, 1985, pp 103–120

Beck JC, van der Kolk B: Reports of childhood incest and current behavior of chronically hospitalized psychotic women. Am J Psychiatry 144:1474–1476, 1987

Blom GE: A school disaster—intervention and research aspects. J Am Acad Child Psychiatry 25:336–345, 1986

Browne A, Finkelhor D: Impact of child sexual abuse: a review of the research. Psychol Bull 99:66–77, 1986

Bryer JB, Nelson BA, Miller JB, et al: Childhood sexual and physical abuse as factors in adult psychiatric illness. Am J Psychiatry 144:1426–1430, 1987

Burgess AW, Hartman CR, McCausland MP, et al: Response patterns in children and adolescents exploited through sex rings and pornography. Am J Psychiatry 141:656–662, 1984

Burgess AW, Hartman CR, McCormack A: Abused to abuser: antecedents of socially deviant behaviors. Am J Psychiatry 144:1431–1436, 1987

Burke JD Jr, Borus JF, Burns BJ, et al: Changes in children's behavior after a natural disaster. Am J Psychiatry 139:1010–1014, 1982

Dollinger SJ: Lightning-strike disaster among children. Br J Med Psychol 58:375–383, 1985

Dollinger SJ, O'Donnell JP, Staley AA: Lightning-strike disaster: effects on children's fears and worries. J Consult Clin Psychol 52:1028–1038, 1984

Earls F, Smith E, Reich W, et al: Investigating psychopathological consequences of a disaster in children: a pilot study incorporating a structured diagnostic interview. J Am Acad Child Adolesc Psychiatry 27:90–95, 1988

Einbender AJ, Friedrich, WN. Psychological functioning and behavior of sexually abused girls. J Consult Clin Psychol 57:155–157, 1989

Eth S, Pynoos RS (eds): Post-Traumatic Stress Disorder in Children. Washington, DC, American Psychiatric Press, 1985

Galante R, Foa D: An epidemiological study of psychic trauma and treatment effectiveness for children after a natural disaster. J Am Acad Child Psychiatry 25:357–363, 1986

Gislason IL, Call JD: Dog bite in infancy: trauma and personality development. J Am Acad Child Psychiatry 21:203–207, 1982

Goldston DB, Turnquist DC, Knutson JF: Presenting problems of sexually abused girls receiving psychiatric services. J Abnorm Psychol 98:314–317, 1989

Gomes-Schwartz B, Horowitz JM, Sauzier M: Severity of emotional distress among sexually abused preschool, school-age, and adolescent children. Hosp Community Psychiatry 36:503–508, 1985

Gould MS, Wunsch-Hitzig R, Dohrenwend B: Estimating the prevalence of childhood psychopathology. J Am Acad Child Psychiatry 20:462–476, 1981

Handford HA, Mayes SD, Mattison RE, et al: Child and parent reaction to the Three Mile Island nuclear accident. J Am Acad Child Psychiatry 25:346–356, 1986

Herman JL, Perry JC, van der Kolk BA: Childhood trauma in borderline personality disorder. Am J Psychiatry 146:490–495, 1989

Kinzie JD, Sack WH, Angell RH, et al: The psychiatric effects of massive trauma on Cambodian children: I. the children. J Am Acad Child Adolesc Psychiatry 25:370–376, 1986

Kinzie JD, Sack W, Angell R, et al: A three-year follow-up of Cambodian young people traumatized as children. J Am Acad Child Adolesc Psychiatry 28:501–504, 1989

Kiser LJ, Ackerman BJ, Brown E, et al: Post-traumatic stress disorder in young children: a reaction to purported sexual abuse. J Am Acad Child Psychiatry 27:645–649, 1988

Kovacs M: The Children's Depression Inventory (CDI). Psychopharmacol Bull 21:995–998, 1985

Krener P: After incest: secondary prevention? J Am Acad Child Psychiatry 24:231–234, 1985

Lindberg FH, Distad LJ: Post-traumatic stress disorders in women who experienced childhood incest. Child Abuse Negl 9:329–334, 1985.

Livingston R: Sexually and physically abused children. J Am Acad Child Adolesc Psychiatry 26:413–415, 1987

Lyons JA: Posttraumatic stress disorder in children and adolescents: a review of the literature. Developmental and Behavioral Pediatrics 8:349–356, 1987

Malmquist CP: Children who witness parental murder: posttraumatic aspects. J Am Acad Child Psychiatry 25:320–325, 1986

Martini DR, Ryan C, Nakayama D, et al: Psychiatric sequelae after traumatic injury: the Pittsburgh Regatta accident. J Am Acad Child Adolesc Psychiatry 29:70–75, 1990

McFarlane AC: Posttraumatic phenomena in a longitudinal study of children following a natural disaster. J Am Acad Child Adolesc Psychiatry 26:764–769, 1987

McFarlane AC: Recent life events and psychiatric disorder in children: the interaction with preceding extreme adversity. J Child Psychol Psychiatry 29:677–690, 1988

McLeer SV, Deblinger E, Atkins MS, et al: Post-traumatic stress disorder in sexually abused children. J Am Acad Child Adolesc Psychiatry 27:650–654, 1988

McNally RJ: Assessment of PTSD in children. Psychological Assessment: A Journal of Consulting and Clinical Psychology 3:531–537, 1991

Milne G: Cyclone Tracy: II the effects on Darwin children. Australian Psychologist 12:55–62, 1977

Newman CJ: Children of disaster: clinical observations at Buffalo Creek. Am J Psychiatry 133:306–312, 1976

Nir Y: Post-traumatic stress disorder in children with cancer, in Post-Traumatic Stress Disorder in Children. Edited by Eth S, Pynoos RS. Washington, DC, American Psychiatric Press, 1985, pp 123–132

Payton JB, Krocker-Tuskan M: Children's reactions to loss of parent through violence. J Am Acad Child Adolesc Psychiatry 27:563–566, 1988

Pynoos RS: Post-traumatic stress disorder in children and adolescents, in Psychiatric Disorders in Children and Adolescents. Edited by Garfinkel BD, Carlson GA, Weller EB. Philadelphia, PA, WB Saunders, 1990, pp 48–63

Pynoos RS, Nader K: Children who witness the sexual assaults of their mothers. J Am Acad Child Adolesc Psychiatry 27:567–572, 1988

Pynoos RS, Frederick C, Nader K, et al: Life threat and posttraumatic stress disorder in school-age children. Arch Gen Psychiatry 44:1057–1063, 1987

Sack WH, Angell RH, Kinzie JD, et al: The psychiatric effects of massive trauma on Cambodian children: II. the family, the home, and the school. J Am Acad Child Adolesc Psychiatry 25:377–383, 1986

Saigh PA: The development and validation of the Children's Posttraumatic Stress Disorder Inventory. International Journal of Special Education 4:75–84, 1989

Saigh PA: The development of posttraumatic stress disorder following four different modes of traumatization. Behav Res Ther 29:213–216, 1991

Sansonnet-Hayden H, Haley G, Marriage K, et al: Sexual abuse and psychopathology in hospitalized adolescents. J Am Acad Child Adolesc Psychiatry 26:753–757, 1987

Schwarz ED, Kowalski JM: Malignant memories: posttraumatic stress disorder in children and adults following a school shooting. J Am Acad Child Adolesc Psychiatry 30:936–944, 1991

Sirles EA, Smith JA, Kusama H: Psychiatric status of intrafamilial child sexual abuse victims. J Am Acad Child Adolesc Psychiatry 28:225–229, 1989

Spitzer RL, Williams JB: Proposed revisions in the DSM-III classification of anxiety disorders based on research and clinical experience, in Anxiety and the Anxiety Disorders. Edited by Tuma AH, Maser JD. Hillsdale, NJ, Erlbaum, 1985, pp 759–774

Stoddard FJ, Norman DK, Murphy JM, et al: Psychiatric outcome of burned children and adolescents. J Am Acad Child Adolesc Psychiatry 28:589–595, 1989

Sugar M: Children in a disaster: an overview. Child Psychiatry Hum Dev 19:163–179, 1989

Terr LC: Children of Chowchilla: a study of psychic trauma. Psychoanal Study Child 34:547–623, 1979

Terr LC: Chowchilla revisited: the effects of psychic trauma four years after a school-bus kidnapping. Am J Psychiatry 140:1543–1550, 1983a

Terr LC: Child snatching: a new epidemic of an ancient malady. J Pediatr 103:151–156, 1983b

Terr LC: Psychic trauma in children and adolescents. Psychiatr Clin North Am 8:815–835, 1985

Welner Z, Reich W, Herjanic B, et al: Reliability, validity, and parent-child agreement studies of the Diagnostic Interview for Children and Adults (DICA). J Am Acad Child Adolesc Psychiatry 26:649–653, 1987

Yule W, Williams RM: Post-traumatic stress reactions in children. Journal of Traumatic Stress 3:279–295, 1990

Ziv A, Israeli R: Effects of bombardment on the manifest anxiety level of children living in kibbutzim. J Consult Clin Psychol 40:287–291, 1973

# ◆ 5 ◆ Disasters and Posttraumatic Stress Disorder

Bonnie L. Green, Ph.D.

***Summary***      This chapter reviews the literature, and on-going research by the author, on traumatic responses to disaster. The information obtained is applied to the question of whether any changes in the present diagnostic criteria for posttraumatic stress disorder (PTSD) are advisable. Studies were reviewed as to type of event, period since disaster, demographic characteristics, number of different experiences and symptoms, gender distribution, interrelationship of symptoms, and areas of omission in the current criteria. The results are discussed, some symptom changes are suggested, and others are endorsed in their present status as in the overall syndrome. A plea is made for better operationalization of existing avoidance criteria.

## Statement of the Issue

This chapter is a review focused on the issue of whether any changes need to be made in the specific symptoms that make up the DSM-III-R (American Psychiatric Association 1987) criteria for PTSD. The general question raised was whether symptoms should be added to or deleted from the criteria set. Data potentially relevant to this issue would include absolute and relative frequencies of the various symptoms within different populations exposed to extreme stressors, as well as internal consistency data for the DSM-III-R symptoms. Further, studies that have addressed a wide variety of stress symptoms in exposed populations might suggest symptoms that are not currently in the criteria that perhaps should be.

The current review was to address these issues with regard to disaster populations, as similar issues were being separately addressed for children

75

(Chapter 4 by McNally), crime victims (Chapter 7 by Kilpatrick and Resnick), and Vietnam War veterans (Chapter 6 by Keane).

Ideally, diagnostic categories should contain a sufficient number of symptoms to allow individuals with the disorder to be identified. Symptoms in the set should be clearly those that apply to most people with the disorder and not those that occur only infrequently or are specific to a particular subset of individuals with the disorder. Symptoms specific to subsets can be noted in the text. Symptoms should be those that differentiate disorders rather than those that overlap among disorders. The symptoms should "hang together" as a syndrome, although it is clear that some symptoms may be alternatives to each other. With these assumptions in mind, PTSD was examined with regard to modification of the specific criteria.

# Method

Studies on disaster were reviewed for the following:

1. Type of event;
2. Period since disaster;
3. Demographic characteristics;
4. Proportions of subjects with various stressor experiences;
5. Proportions of subjects with various PTSD symptoms (either DSM-III [American Psychiatric Association 1980] or DSM-III-R);
6. Gender-related distribution of PTSD;
7. Interrelationship of PTSD symptoms; and
8. The issue of stress symptoms that are not addressed in the criteria.

# Results

## Availability of Information

The availability of information on the topic addressed was disappointing. Information was extremely sparse. A number of studies were indeed located but were based on DSM-III criteria. The time lag between the establishment of the DSM-III-R criteria and the present revision is simply too short to have allowed for studies using DSM-III-R to be designed, submitted for funding, implemented, written up, and published at this writing. Some authors collecting clinical data on an ongoing basis may have had time for this turnaround, or possibly those researchers just going into the field who could revise criteria at the last moment. However, no research in the area of disaster could be located. A study from my own research group is included that was based on a draft of DSM-III-R so that it contains most of the symptoms of the present criteria, but not all.

Quite a few studies were located that used the Diagnostic Interview Schedule—Disaster Supplement (DIS-DS) to measure most (although not all) symptoms of DSM-III (Robins and Smith 1983).

These studies are the most comparable. In no case was internal consistency data reported for the samples, either for the overall diagnosis or for the separate classes of criteria.

## Symptom Frequencies and Interrelationships

Table 5–1 shows the five studies located that contained PTSD symptom data at six data collection points. The studies are organized by time, with the studies closer in time to the traumatic event on the left and those farther away on the right. Both rank order or symptom and actual percentage of the study sample having the symptom are presented. Symptoms are organized by DSM-III-R categories even though the studies were all based on DSM-III. It is clear that there is wide variation in the absolute levels of symptoms from one study to the next. Because the instrument used to gather the data was the same in each case, the differences cannot presumably be attributed to method variance. However, because the disasters as well as the time periods and sites varied, it is impossible to disentangle main effects. The highest level of symptoms was found in the acute phase following a jet crash (Smith and North 1988).

Two other studies were located that reported on DSM-III symptoms that are not included in the table: Wilkinson's (1983) study of the Hyatt Regency skywalk collapse in Kansas City, Missouri, and Madakasira and O'Brien's (1987) study of a tornado in North Carolina. The latter study used a self-report checklist to gather data rather than a structured interview; in the former, the exact mode of data collection was not clear. In both cases the rates of PTSD symptoms were much higher than in the studies using the DIS.

Of most salience to the present report, the *relative* frequency of symptoms within study was noted to ascertain whether there were any patterns with regard to which symptoms occurred most often and which were rela-

Table 5–1.  Rank order (and percentage) of PTSD symptoms in several studies using the DIS-DS to rate DSM-III symptoms

| Time Period | 1 Month | 1–1½ Months | 2–4 Months | 3–4 Months* | 12 Months | 16 Months* | x̄ Rank |
|---|---|---|---|---|---|---|---|
| Disaster | Tornado | Jet Crash | Fire | Flood | Dioxin/ Flood | Flood | |
| Investigator | North et al. 1989 | Smith and North 1988 | Maida et al. 1989 | Steinglass and Gerrity 1990 | Canino and Solomon 1990 | Steinglass and Gerrity 1990 | |
| B) Nightmares or remembering | 5 (17) | 1 (72) | 4.5 (12) | 2 (45) | 1 (11) | 2 (15) | 2.6 |
| Happening again | 6.5 (10) | 7 (33) | 6 (8) | 5 (23) | 4 (4) | 8 (3) | 6.1 |
| Problems worse with reminders | 5 (21) | 5.5 (48) | — | 7 (21) | 2.5 (6) | 3 (13) | 4.6 |
| C) Avoid activities that remind | 6.5 (10) | 3.5 (50) | 3 (16) | 8 (20) | 6.5 (2) | 5.5 (11) | 5.5 |
| Loss of interest or caring | 9 (2) | 9 (24) | 7 (4) | 6 (22) | 5.5 (2) | 1 (17) | 6.3 |
| D) Trouble sleeping | 1 (31) | 2 (65) | 1 (32) | 1 (63) | 2.5 (6) | 4 (12) | 1.9 |
| Trouble concentrating | 2.5 (29) | 5.5 (48) | 4.5 (12) | 3 (42) | 8 (1) | 5.5 (11) | 4.8 |
| Jumping/easily startled | 2.5 (29) | 3.5 (50) | 2 (24) | 4 (24) | 5 (3) | 7 (6) | 4.0 |
| Ashamed of being alive | 8 (7) | 8 (28) | 8 (0) | 9 (3) | — | 9 (2) | 8.4 |

* Figures were reported for men and women separately.  Approximate averages were used for this table.

tively infrequent. It should be noted that the DIS combined some symptoms in the DSM-III criteria (Robins and Smith 1983, pp 72–84). Repetitive intrusive recollections and repetitive dreams are combined into one item asking about experiences that caused the subject "nightmares or (to) keep remembering the experience." All of the "C" symptoms were combined into one item: "loss of the ability to care about others or loss of interest in things you previously enjoyed." Avoidance of activities or situations that remind the person of the event is currently a "C" symptom. Survivor guilt in the DIS is operationalized by a question asking about a horrifying experience that made the subject feel "ashamed of still being alive."

Although there is some variability in rank across the studies, there is some range in the relative frequency of symptoms. The two most frequent symptoms were "trouble sleeping" and "nightmares/remembering." The least frequent symptom was "ashamed of being alive." "Jumpy/easily startled" was somewhat more frequent while "loss of interest or caring" and feeling that the experience was happening again were relatively less frequent. Rank did not appear to be associated with elapsed time since event.

Rank order or symptoms in a study with a much later follow-up period can be found in Table 5–2 (survivors of the Buffalo Creek, West Virginia, dam disaster 14 years postevent). That study used draft DSM-III-R criteria and the information was collected using the Structured Clinical Interview for DSM-III-R (SCID). At 14 years postevent, the most frequent current symptoms reported by the subjects were avoidance of thoughts of the event and psychological distress at reminders. Intrusive thoughts and repetitive dreams had very different relative frequencies, suggesting the importance of measuring these separately. Intrusive thoughts were relatively common, whereas dreams of the event were uncommon. The least common symptoms were numbing, irritability, and flashbacks. Survivor guilt (not a formal criterion in DSM-III-R) occurred in about 15% of the subjects.

Similarities between the two types of data (DIS-DS, early and SCID, late) seem to be the infrequency of guilt or shame and to some extent of numbing/not caring as a symptom. Conversely, dreams/nightmares, recollections, and sleep difficulties are relatively common symptoms. Avoidance of thoughts about the event, not measured in the DIS-DS, was the *most* common symptom among Buffalo Creek survivors.

Tables 5–3 and 5–4 contain intercorrelations among PTSD symptoms for two studies (Green et al. 1990b; S. D. Solomon, unpublished data, Jan-

Table 5–2.   Current PTSD symptoms in a second-decade sample: Buffalo Creek Dam collapse (14 years postevent; $N = 96$ with complete data)

| | % With Symptom | Rank | Met Criteria |
|---|---|---|---|
| B. Intrusive thoughts | 48 | 3 | |
| Dreams or nightmares | 23 | 11 | |
| Flashbacks | 19 | 13 | |
| Distress (psychological or physiological) at reminders | 50 | 2 | |
| | | | B/65% |
| C. Avoid thoughts | 52 | 1 | |
| Avoid activities | 40 | 6 | |
| Amnesia | 22 | 12 | |
| Loss of interest | 31 | 9 | |
| Detached/estranged | 26 | 10 | |
| Numbing of feelings | 15 | 15 | |
| Foreshortened future | — | | |
| | | | C/49% |
| D. Trouble sleeping | 45 | 4 | |
| Irritable | 17 | 14 | |
| Trouble concentrating | 35 | 8 | |
| Hypervigilance | 37 | 7 | |
| Jumpy/easily startled | 44 | 5 | |
| Physiological reaction to exposure | — | | |
| | | | D/64% |
| PTSD/current | | | PTSD/25% |

uary 1990). The former is at 1 month postexposure (with relatively similar figures at 12 months) for DSM-III symptoms, whereas the latter is at 14 years postexposure with DSM-III-R symptoms. The symptoms are clearly interrelated to a significant extent. The DSM-III symptoms seem somewhat more highly interrelated. This could be due to a variety of factors, including time, type of event, and instrument used (e.g., the DIS requires that the subject link the symptom with a particular "horrifying" event). Internal consistencies (coefficient alpha) for the Buffalo Creek study were .57 for B (intrusion) symptoms, .81 for C (denial) symptoms, .78 for hyperarousal (D) symptoms, and .86 for the PTSD diagnosis (all symptoms).

## Gender Ratios

Several of the studies reported on PTSD rates separately by gender. The findings were mixed. Smith and North (1988) and Madakasira and O'Brien (1987) reported no differences between genders in the rates of

**Table 5–3.** Intercorrelations among PTSD symptoms at 1 month (DIS)—St. Louis dioxin study

| | Nightmares/ Remembering | Happening Again | Symptoms Worse | Avoid Activities | Loss of Interest | Sleep | Concentration | Startle |
|---|---|---|---|---|---|---|---|---|
| B) Nightmares/ Remembering | | 55 | 70 | 36 | 42 | 70 | 21 | 51 |
| Happening again | | | 43 | 42 | 17 | 31 | 37 | 28 |
| Symptoms worse at exposure | | | | 15 | 59 | 52 | -0.2 | 73 |
| C) Avoid activities | | | | | 28 | 33 | 57 | 22 |
| Loss of interest | | | | | | 43 | -01 | 60 |
| D) Sleep | | | | | | | 29 | 34 |
| Concentration | | | | | | | | -01 |
| Startle | | | | | | | | |

**Table 5–4.** Intercorrelations among PTSD symptoms in a second decade sample (SCID)—Buffalo Creek study

| | | B1 | B2 | B3 | B4 | C1 | C2 | C3 | C4 | C5 | C6 | D1 | D2 | D3 | D4 | D5 | PTSD |
|---|---|---|---|---|---|---|---|---|---|---|---|---|---|---|---|---|---|
| B1 | Intrusions | | 33 | 13 | 39 | 42 | 15 | 23 | 31 | 22 | 17 | 18 | 04 | 23 | 28 | 27 | 33 |
| B2 | Dreams | | | 16 | 13 | 12 | 12 | 06 | 15 | 13 | 14 | 13 | 30 | 16 | 38 | 16 | 38 |
| B3 | Flashbacks | | | | 35 | 27 | 40 | 26 | 43 | 34 | 47 | 20 | 15 | 41 | 01 | 13 | 35 |
| B4 | Reactivity | | | | | 36 | 40 | 09 | 36 | 34 | 34 | 40 | 29 | 34 | 20 | 23 | 33 |
| C1 | Avoid thoughts | | | | | | 56 | 33 | 52 | 45 | 33 | 33 | 13 | 26 | 29 | 35 | 38 |
| C2 | Avoid reminders | | | | | | | 43 | 39 | 29 | 37 | 35 | 10 | 31 | 19 | 30 | 34 |
| C3 | Amnesia | | | | | | | | 28 | 07 | 28 | 34 | 07 | 26 | 22 | 23 | 33 |
| C4 | Less interest | | | | | | | | | 63 | 64 | 36 | 27 | 52 | 34 | 26 | 49 |
| C5 | Detaching | | | | | | | | | | 53 | 25 | 32 | 47 | 15 | 23 | 39 |
| C6 | Numbing | | | | | | | | | | | 28 | 32 | 53 | 09 | 32 | 39 |
| D1 | Trouble sleeping | | | | | | | | | | | | 38 | 61 | 38 | 34 | 45 |
| D2 | Irritable | | | | | | | | | | | | | 44 | 38 | 36 | 43 |
| D3 | Trouble concentrating | | | | | | | | | | | | | | 36 | 31 | 54 |
| D4 | Hypervigilance | | | | | | | | | | | | | | | 39 | 50 |
| D5 | Jumpy/startled | | | | | | | | | | | | | | | | 39 |

PTSD following a jet crash and a tornado, respectively. On the other hand, Steinglass and Gerrity's study (1990) of a West Virginia flood showed higher rates of PTSD and PTSD symptoms for women (8 of 11 cases of PTSD at 4 months were women). Wilkinson (1983) showed more frequent symptoms of sleep disturbance and difficulty concentrating in women than in men, and our Buffalo Creek follow-up study (Green et al. 1990b) showed higher PTSD rates for women than men at both 2 years (52% versus 32%) and 14 years postevent (31% versus 23%).

## Related Symptoms

A further area of exploration was symptoms that might not be found in the criteria but would be highly associated with PTSD symptoms and should perhaps be considered as possible additions to the criteria or to the text. On the one hand, this issue has been addressed very broadly in studies that measure a variety of symptoms but not usually PTSD. On the other hand, studies that have focused on PTSD symptoms have tended not to examine other symptoms so that the relative importance of noncriteria symptoms cannot be determined. Thus this issue is quite difficult to address. Further, since this was a secondary issue to the mandate of this chapter, it was not addressed comprehensively. If searching the literature for articles on specific PTSD symptoms was difficult, searching for articles on missing symptoms was essentially impossible. Thus, reliance was placed on studies located for other purposes and reviewed for mention of prominent symptoms that might not be part of the criteria. Few authors addressed this issue.

Further, a study under way by my research team recently addressed a related issue (i.e., whether stress symptoms differed by type of disaster). A small portion of those data will be presented here as being relevant to the general question.

Smith and North (1988) showed more new cases of a diagnosis of depression following the Ramada jet crash in Indianapolis than new PTSD cases. There were also new cases of generalized anxiety disorder (GAD) and some symptoms of depression following the Baldwin Hills fire in Los Angeles. Wilkinson (1983) found high rates of sadness, fatigue, recurrent anxiety and depression, decreased appetite, and decreased enthusiasm following the Hyatt skywalk collapse. Madakasira and O'Brien (1987) found decreased libido in one-third of their subjects following a tornado in North Carolina, as well as a high incidence of memory impairment. Symptom Checklist scales correlating with PTSD were those for depression and somatization.

Our own group took a somewhat different approach (Green et al. 1989a, 1989b). We combined data sets from four disaster studies and examined clinically rated and self-reported symptom scales or clusters that we showed empirically to be related to stressor experiences (specifically life threat, loss of loved one, and exposure to grotesque death). Four studies were used: 1) the Beverly Hills Supper Club study 1 year postevent (Green et al. 1985), 2) the Buffalo Creek dam collapse study 2 years postevent (Gleser et al. 1981), 3) the Vietnam veteran study an average of 10–15 years postevent (Green et al. 1990a), and 4) the Buffalo Creek follow-up study 14 years postevent (Green et al. 1990b). Clinical ratings were made on the Psychiatric Evaluation Form (PEF; Endicott and Spitzer 1972) and the self-report items were selected from the Symptom Checklist-90 (SCL-90; Derogatis 1983) plus 12 items covering specific PTSD symptoms. The 80 items in the Cincinnati Stress Response Schedule (CSRS; B. L. Green, unpublished data, October 1990) were those that correlated with the stressor variables at or above .25. These 80 items were then factor-analyzed and seven clusters were obtained (see Table 5–5).

**Table 5–5.** Factors for the Cincinnati Stress Response Schedule (CSRS)

| SCL Item Number | Core PTSD Cluster |
| --- | --- |
| 2. | Nervousness or shakiness inside |
| 3. | Unwanted thoughts, words, or ideas that won't leave your mind |
| 11. | Feeling easily annoyed or irritated |
| 22. | Feeling of being trapped or caught |
| 26. | Blaming yourself for things |
| 28. | Feeling blocked in getting things done |
| 29. | Felling lonely |
| 30. | Feeling blue |
| 31. | Worrying too much about things |
| 32. | Feeling no interest in things |
| 34. | Your feelings being easily hurt |
| 36. | Feeling others do not understand you or are unsympathetic |
| 41. | Feeling inferior to others |
| 46. | Difficulty making decisions |
| 57. | Feeling tense or keyed up |
| 69. | Feeling very self-conscious with others |
| 77. | Feeling lonely even when you are with people |
| 78. | Feeling so restless you couldn't sit still |
| 79. | Feelings of worthlessness |
| 92. | Frightening dreams or nightmares |
| 94. | Feeling jumpy or easily startled |

| SCL Item Number | Sleep Disturbance |
| --- | --- |
| 44. | Trouble falling asleep |
| 64. | Awakening in the early morning |
| 66. | Sleep that is restless or disturbed |

| SCL ItemNumber | Phobic Avoidance |
| --- | --- |
| 13. | Feeling afraid in open spaces or on the streets |
| 23. | Suddenly scared for no reason |
| 25. | Feeling afraid to go out of your house alone |
| 33. | Feeling fearful |
| 47. | Feeling afraid to travel on buses, subways, or trains |
| 50. | Having to avoid certain things, places, or activities because they frighten you |
| 70. | Feeling uneasy in crowds, such as shopping or at a movie |
| 72. | Spells of fear or panic |
| 73. | Feeling uncomfortable about eating or drinking in public |
| 75. | Feeling nervous when you are left alone |
| 96. | Images that intrude unexpectedly |

| SCL Item Number | Obsessive-Compulsive |
| --- | --- |
| 9. | Trouble remembering things |
| 38. | Having to do things very slowly to insure correctness |
| 45. | Having to check and double check what you do |
| 51. | Your mind going blank |
| 55. | Trouble concentrating |
| 65. | Having to repeat the same actions such as touching, counting, washing |

**Table 5–5.** Factors for the Cincinnati Stress Response Schedule (CSRS) (continued)

| SCL Item Number | Paranoid |
| --- | --- |
| 7. | The idea that someone else can control your thoughts |
| 16. | Hearing voices that other people do not hear |
| 18. | Feeling that most people cannot be trusted |
| 35. | Other people being aware of your private thoughts |
| 37. | Feeling that people are unfriendly or dislike you |
| 83. | Feeling that people will take advantage of you if you let them |
| 97. | The inability to trust others |

| SCL ItemNumber | Somatic |
| --- | --- |
| 1. | Headaches |
| 4. | Faintness or dizziness |
| 12. | Pains in heart or chest |
| 14. | Feeling low in energy or slowed down |
| 17. | Trembling |
| 39. | Heart pounding or racing |
| 40. | Nausea or upset stomach |
| 42. | Soreness of your muscles |
| 48. | Trouble getting your breath |
| 49. | Hot or cold spells |
| 52. | Numbness or tingling in parts of your body |
| 53. | A lump in your throat |
| 56. | Feeling weak in parts of your body |
| 58. | Heavy feelings in your arms or legs |
| 71. | Feeling everything is an effort |
| 87. | The idea that something serious is wrong with your body |

| SCL Item Number | Borderline |
| --- | --- |
| 15. | Thoughts of ending your life |
| 24. | Temper outbursts that you could not control |
| 59. | Thoughts of death or dying |
| 63. | Having urges to beat, injure, or harm someone |
| 67. | Having urges to break or smash things |
| 68. | Having ideas or feelings that others do not share |
| 80. | Feeling that familiar things are strange or unreal |
| 81. | Shouting or throwing things |
| 86. | The idea that you should be punished for your sins |
| 88. | Never feeling close to another person |
| 89. | Feelings of guilt |
| 90. | The idea that something is wrong with your mind |
| 93. | The feeling that you are losing control |
| 95. | Thoughts of how you might die |
| 98. | The feeling that your life has no meaning |
| 100. | The feeling that you are to blame or are responsible for things that happen to other people |

The largest cluster (21 items) we labeled *Core PTSD* because it included a variety of items occurring across the three DSM-III-R PTSD criteria sets (i.e., intrusion, denial, arousal): frightening dreams and nightmares, feeling no interest in things, and feeling easily annoyed or irritated. This cluster included typical depression and anxiety symptoms as well. The *Sleep Disturbance* cluster included all of the sleep problems in the original inventory of items. *Phobic Avoidance* overlapped a great deal with the "Phobic Anxiety" scale on the SCL-90 and included fear of a variety of situations (e.g., travel, open spaces, being alone) and avoidance of or discomfort with certain activities. These first three clusters we viewed as central to the stress response and expected that they would be elevated in all groups of survivors. The four additional clusters (see next paragraph) included symptoms that are not included in the PTSD criteria. We hypothesized that they would be less frequent and more likely to vary by type of trauma or group.

The *Obsessive-Compulsive* cluster overlapped somewhat with the SCL-90 cluster of the same name and included repetitive acts and trouble concentrating. *Paranoid* symptoms covered primarily issues of trust, along with some more psychotic-type symptoms (hearing voices that others cannot hear) that may reflect intrusive phenomena. The *Somatic* cluster overlapped a fair amount, although not completely, with the "Somatization" scale on the SCL-90. Our cluster also included additional physical aspects of anxiety and depression. Finally, the *Borderline* cluster contained a range of symptoms that were somewhat difficult to name. The symptoms included hostility, guilt, thoughts of death and suicide, uncontrollable temper, and not feeling close to others. These items seemed best united under a diagnostic term that encompasses this range of symptoms.

For purposes of the current report, only the profiles for the two samples on whom we had diagnostic information are presented (the Buffalo Creek 14-year follow-up sample and the Vietnam veteran sample). Figure 5–1 shows the profiles for those subjects with a PTSD diagnosis in each sample for the clinical (PEF) ratings. It can be seen that the profiles are fairly similar, with anxiety and depression ratings being relatively high. For the Vietnam veterans, social isolation was the highest rating; this particular symptom was much lower in the Buffalo Creek sample. Although the remaining ratings were relatively lower, the veterans were still notably higher than Buffalo Creek residents on suspicion, belligerence, and alcohol abuse. Their overall level of impairment was quite similar (3.0 versus 2.8). The Buffalo Creek

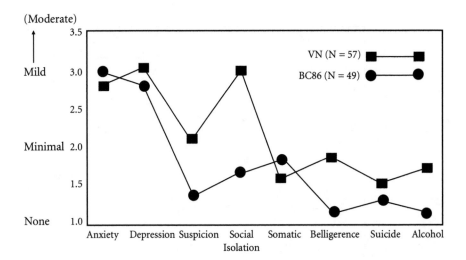

**Figure 5–1.**   PEF profiles on selected scales for two second-decade groups with PTSD (raw scores). VN = Vietnam veteran study; BC86 = Buffalo Creek 14-year postevent study.

survivors, on the other hand, were somewhat higher on somatic complaints (as well as anxiety).

Turning to the self-reported symptoms in the CSRS (Figure 5–2), again the profiles look similar, with *Sleep Disturbance* showing the highest ratings for both groups. In the veterans, this was followed by "core" symptoms and then by *Borderline* symptoms. For Buffalo Creek survivors, "core" symptoms, obsessive-compulsive symptoms, and somatic symptoms were prominent.

Using only the civilian samples, men and women were compared on both instruments, and differences were found to be quite minimal. Profiles were essentially the same, with women having slightly more anxiety and men having slightly more alcohol abuse.

High comorbidity was found in both samples with major depression and GAD. In the Vietnam veteran study, fairly high overlap was also seen with panic and phobic disorders.

## Relationship of PTSD Symptoms to Stressors

The data just presented were also examined by type of stressor experience. Specifically, profiles of individuals who experienced life threat in these three events (Buffalo Creek, Beverly Hills, Vietnam) were compared with

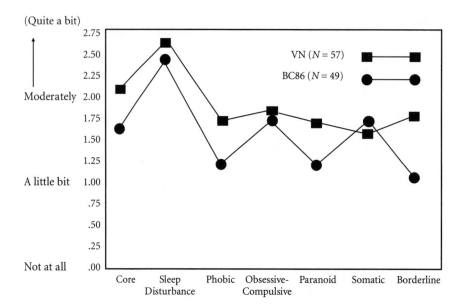

**Figure 5–2.** CSRS profiles on seven clusters for two second-decade groups with PTSD (raw scores). VN = Vietnam veteran study; BC86 = Buffalo Creek 14-year postevent study.

individuals who experienced loss of a friend or relative, and those who witnessed grotesque or mutilating deaths. Although there was some over-lap among these groups, the correlations among the three stressors were actually quite low, ranging from .18 to .27. Figures 5–3 and 5–4 show the results of this comparison. The profiles are strikingly similar for the three different types of stressors, suggesting that these various aspects of the stressor experiences produce similar types of symptoms.

Finally, specific stressor experiences were correlated with the individual PTSD symptoms from the Buffalo Creek follow-up study to assess the level of association between specific experiences and symptoms at 14 years postevent. Although the overall diagnosis of current PTSD at 14 years was associated with a number of specific experiences (loss of a household mem-ber, prolonged exposure to the elements, being blocked in one's escape from the flood waters, and being injured), individual symptoms and aspects of the dam collapse showed generally weak relationships.

The only intrusive symptom linked with specific experiences was recur-rent dreams; these occurred more often to people who lost valuable posses-sions in the dam collapse and to those who lost a member of their household. Criterion C5, detachment, was associated only with seeing the dead bodies of individuals known to the subject. Hyperarousal symptoms were much more often associated with specific stressors. Sleep disturbance was predicted by seeing and/or identifying dead bodies, difficulty concentrating was associated with identifying bodies and/or seeing the bodies of

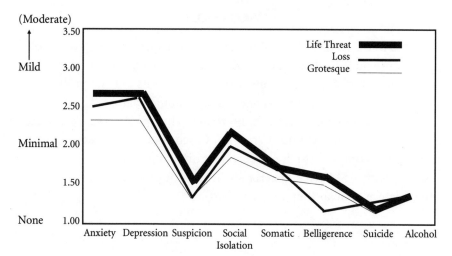

**Figure 5–3.**  PEF profiles of selected scales for three risk groups (raw scores); $N = 368$.

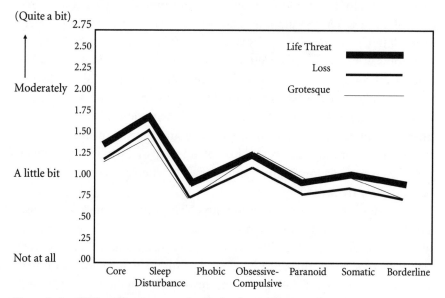

**Figure 5–4.**  CSRS profiles on seven clusters for three risk groups (raw scores); $N = 240$.

people known to the subject, and hypervigilance was associated with actually being *in* the flood waters as they raged down the valley and with loss of immediate family. All correlations were in the mid .20s or low .30s and thus explained only a small portion of variance in the symptom reports.

# Discussion

As noted in the results, the findings from this chapter are *extremely* modest, because published data on PTSD symptoms using DSM-III-R criteria with regard to disasters are nonexistent. This points out the problem of undertaking frequent revisions of diagnostic nomenclature. The problem of lack of information is particularly crucial to the question under investigation (i.e., specific symptom criteria). Given these difficulties, my current report is only able to draw broad tentative conclusions pending more research with DSM-III-R criteria in the area of disasters (which may be out of date as soon as they are published).

## Symptom Prevalence

The purpose of examining the symptom criteria separately for their occurrence was to determine whether any symptoms were particularly important in disaster populations and whether any seemed particularly irrelevant. Using the DIS-DS was problematic, because even DSM-III symptoms were combined or left out. The most frequent symptoms using that methodology were "nightmares/remembering" and "sleep disturbance," while "ashamed of being alive" was quite infrequent. The Buffalo Creek data using the SCID at a much later time period distinguished intrusive thoughts from dreams or nightmares and showed the former to be much more common. However, loss of interest or caring and survivor guilt were relatively low in that sample as well, whereas sleep disturbance was relatively frequent.

These findings are actually compatible. The Buffalo Creek study also measured avoidance symptoms not picked up in the DIS-DS and showed avoidance of thoughts about the event to be quite common. The relatively high level of sleep disturbance in all studies supports the contention that sleep disorder is a significant symptom. However, it is not invariably present in community samples. Frequencies in the samples reviewed here ranged from 6% in the St. Louis dioxin study to 65% closely following the Ramada jet crash. Clinical populations would undoubtedly show higher levels.

Currently, DSM-III-R requires at least three out of seven avoidance symptoms (Criterion C) for the diagnosis of PTSD. Some concern has been expressed that this is excessive. For example, studies by Solomon and Canino (1990) and Creamer's (1989) study of urban shooting victims all showed low levels of avoidance symptoms. These may, in part, be due to use of the DIS, which may underestimate the denial criteria (see Chapter 1 by Blank and Chapter 8 by Davidson and Fairbank for further discussion of the DIS). Nevertheless, it is also possible that the increased sense of communal identity following a disaster may make the avoidance of social relationships less likely, at least in time periods close to the event.

We examined the frequency of avoidance symptoms in the Buffalo Creek sample, which was not confounded by limitations of the DIS. In that study, every subject had been through the flood and was therefore defined as meeting the "A" criterion (although individual experiences were also assessed). The SCID does not require the subject to link all of the "C" symptoms to the traumatic event. Even so, amnesia and numbing symptoms were quite infrequent. Also, our instrument was based on the second draft of DSM-III-R criteria and did not include "foreshortened future." However, it is not clear exactly how this variable would be operationalized for adults (examples are given for children). We tried to assess it in our Buffalo Creek study (although it was not in the criteria) by having subjects from the experimental and comparison samples mark on a time line between birth and death where they presently were located. Controlling for age, there were no differences between the groups in the extent to which they projected themselves into the future using this metaphor.

This symptom was added at the last minute to DSM-III-R because it was thought to be applicable to children. At the same time (i.e., subsequent to the final meeting of the committee) an arbitrary decision was made to require three rather than two "C" symptoms. Given the questions that have been raised about the scarcity of "C" symptoms, the difficulty of subjects in reporting on these (e.g., ones feelings of numbness, how one has "forgotten" something) and the difficulty in agreeing on an operationalization of some of these symptoms (particularly foreshortened future), argument is made that only two of the symptoms be required to meet the C criterion of the diagnosis rather than the three symptoms currently required. This would allow people who were primarily in an "avoidant" mode to meet the criteria (C [1] and [2]) as well as those who were primarily in a "numbing" mode (C [4]–[6]). The more esoteric symptoms (amnesia, foreshortened future) would help catch cases that were not as clear-cut but would not be required for more routine and perhaps more mild cases.

Survivor guilt, at least as measured by the DIS, where it is operationalized somewhat strangely, does seem infrequent and its removal from the DSM-III-R criteria would appear justified. Even in the Buffalo Creek flood, where many people (friends and neighbors) died and where survivor guilt was operationalized in the SCID by questions about whether the person wondered about surviving when others did not and about any of his or her behaviors during the event that were worrisome, it was still quite infrequent (if ranked, it would have tied for last place).

Internal consistency in the Buffalo Creek data was relatively high for the diagnosis as a whole (.86 for PTSD) and somewhat lower for the separate criteria sets. It was the lowest (.57) for intrusive phenomena. The DIS intercorrelations imply that intrusions would have been more internally consistent in that study. However, the overall figures are quite reasonable evidence for a "syndrome," especially when some symptoms are likely to be alternatives to each other and therefore not necessarily extremely highly correlated.

## Gender Ratios

The evidence on gender ratios is quite mixed, but several clinical and epidemiological studies show a preponderance of the diagnosis in women. One barrier to examining this issue in clinical, or "at-risk" populations, is that a number of investigators focus on survivors of one sex (e.g., Vietnam War veterans, usually men, or rape or incest victims, usually women). Investigators studying disasters or crime should be able to address this question. Higher rates for women have been found in a number of epidemiological studies (Breslau et al. 1991; Davidson et al. 1991; Helzer et al. 1987) and are consistent with other Epidemiologic Catchment Area (ECA) data for anxiety and depression (Myers et al. 1984).

## Related Symptoms

Related symptoms are a particularly difficult problem, because the question has not been studied systematically. It is clear that high comorbidity exists with symptoms of anxiety and depression. In some cases, rates of depression are higher than rates of PTSD following traumatic experiences. One reason for this phenomenon may be simply the overlap between PTSD symptoms and symptoms for depression and anxiety disorder. Although it is clear that general anxiety and depression often accompany PTSD, adding them to the criteria will only increase the overlap problems and make PTSD even less distinct than it already is.

However, in the data presented from our group's study of several disaster/trauma populations, somatic symptoms emerged as being relatively important in the PTSD groups. These symptoms were not necessarily those associated with hyperarousal, but more common complaints such as headache, upset stomach, and so on. Kuhne and colleagues (1988) also found the link between somatization and/or hypochondriacal fixation and PTSD in their sample of substance abusing veterans. Penk and colleagues (1981) had similar findings. Madakasira and O'Brien (1987) found PTSD to be correlated with somatization. The epidemiological findings regarding PTSD and somatization disorder have already been described (see Chapter 8 by Davidson and Fairbank). Because psychosomatic and hypochondriacal symptoms have classically been considered part of the phenomenology of "traumatic neurosis," they should perhaps be considered for inclusion in the PTSD criteria. Although there is probably not enough evidence to make this change for DSM-IV, investigators should more routinely include assessments of this area in their studies so that more evidence is forthcoming.

## PTSD Symptoms and Stressors

No published data were identified linking specific PTSD symptoms with different aspects of stressor experiences. There is clear-cut evidence that the PTSD diagnosis is related to the intensity and frequency of traumatic experiences and to a variety of types of experiences (e.g., Green 1990). However, data by symptoms have not been available. The unpublished data from our Buffalo Creek 14-year follow-up study are interesting in this regard although certainly not ideal. Even if one assumes that early PTSD symptoms are intimately connected to the nature and the intensity of the traumatic events, the maintenance of specific symptoms over years and even decades is likely to be multiply determined; therefore, one would not necessarily expect high links for all symptoms. Only dreams, detachment, sleep disturbance, and difficulty concentrating were associated with particular aspects of the flood experience.

It is interesting that the links, though weak, cut across all three of the criteria sets (B, C, and D). Individual differences, in addition to being mediated by other individual factors, may also be overshadowed by commonalities in experiences among survivors. In any case, some subset of symptoms in the three categories are related to stressor experiences based on one study of long-term follow-up. Clearly more work is needed before discussions about symptom inclusion or exclusion can be informed by specific links of the symptoms with stressors.

The similarity of profiles between subjects with different generic stressor experiences (loss, life threat, exposure to grotesque death) was actually quite surprising given the differences in profiles between types of disaster. These findings imply that some of the differences in profile between traumatized groups may be due to differences in individual characteristics of the groups that were exposed to the various events (e.g., age, culture) rather than the nature of their experiences. Even though life threat and violent and sudden loss are conceptually quite distinct, they may well evoke some of the same associations, thoughts, and vulnerabilities. Both are likely to lead to one's confrontation with unexpected death and the feeling of vulnerability that such confrontation is likely to produce. Exposure to grotesque death, which is somewhat different (i.e., more indirect), may still confront the individual with the real possibility of death in a way that the person could have denied prior to the event. This does imply a common thread of exposure to death across the various types of experiences within events. It would be desirable for investigators to continue to examine how individual experiences affect the particular symptom picture across the wide range of disasters, whether or not individuals meet the full criteria for PTSD.

## Conclusions and Recommendations

Based on the sparsity of the data base, few recommendations can be made in favor of changing the symptomatology of PTSD. Data simply were not available for DSM-III-R by separate symptoms. As a result, this review was based largely on DSM-III criteria, unpublished data from one study using DSM-III-R, and related research on symptoms across trauma groups by my own research team.

The scant evidence suggests that PTSD symptoms "hang together" fairly well and do indeed seem to constitute a syndrome. The least common symptoms are survivor guilt (which is no longer in the criteria) and some of the denial ("C") symptoms.

Not enough evidence has accumulated to drop any of the symptoms. However, it is suggested that only two symptoms be required to meet the "C" criteria until more evidence suggests otherwise. The current requirement of "3 from column C" may artificially reduce the number of people who receive the diagnosis. At the same time, a great deal of attention needs to be given to the instruments used to collect the data. The issue of the subject having to make the link between trauma and symptoms him- or herself is important. But it is also important to consider the issue of how certain criteria are operationalized both conceptually (i.e., what is it we are really looking for?) and in terms of how questions are asked of research subjects/clinical patients. It is one thing for a clinician to listen to a patient for many hours and surmise that the person does not project him- or herself in the future the way other patients do. It is quite another to devise a question that can assess this in 1 or 2 minutes in a structured interview (e.g., the "foreshortened future" question in the SCID: "Did you notice a change in the way you think about or plan for the future?"). If these latter methodologic ideas are addressed more carefully, the substantive issues should be easier to tackle.

Self-report data were de-emphasized throughout this review. The two studies using self-report to assess PTSD had much higher symptom levels. Although this is becoming a more common practice, we actually know very little about the relationship between structured interviews and symptom checklists and about the adequacy of the latter to assess diagnosis. This issue should be studied more systematically. It is relevant to all of DSM-IV, not just PTSD.

There was some hint in the data sources that PTSD is more common in women than in men. There was also a hint that somatic symptoms are an important but unacknowledged aspect of PTSD. Although the evidence is probably not strong enough at present to change the DSM-IV criteria or the text, both of these issues are highlighted as needing research in the near future.

More attention should also be given in the future to linking specific symptoms with aspects of the stressor experience. Because PTSD is a disorder with a specified etiology (meaning that the traumatic experience is necessary for the diagnosis, if not sufficient), the symptoms should be able to be linked with the intensity or frequency aspects of the traumatic experience. Such studies may be difficult to do within study populations where survivors have had similar experiences. However, such data should be available from community samples where the range of experiences is broad.

# References

American Psychiatric Association: Diagnostic and Statistical Manual of Mental Disorders, 3rd Edition. Washington, DC, American Psychiatric Association, 1980

American Psychiatric Association: Diagnostic and Statistical Manual of Mental Disorders, 3rd Edition, Revised. Washington, DC, American Psychiatric Association, 1987

Breslau N, Davis GC, Andreski P: Traumatic events and post-traumatic stress disorder in an urban population of young adults. Arch Gen Psychiatry 48:216–222, 1991

Creamer M: Post-traumatic stress disorder: some diagnostic and clinical issues. Aust N Z J Psychiatry 23:517–522, 1989

Davidson JRT, Hughes D, Blazer DG, et al: Posttraumatic stress disorder in the community: an epidemiological study. Psychol Med 21:1–9, 1991

Derogatis LR: SCL-90 R Version Manual I. Baltimore, MD, Johns Hopkins University Press, 1983

Endicott J, Spitzer RL: What! Another rating scale? The Psychiatric Evaluation Form. J Nerv Ment Dis 154:88–104, 1972

Gleser CG, Green BL, Winger CN: Prolonged Psychosocial Effects of Disaster: A Study of Buffalo Creek. New York, Academic Press, 1981

Green BL: Defining trauma: Terminology and generic stressor dimensions. Journal of Applied Social Psychology 20:1632–1642, 1990

Green BL, Grace MC, Gleser CG: Identifying survivors at risk: long term impairment following the Beverly Hills Supper Club fire. J Consult Clin Psychol 53:672–678, 1985

Green BL, Grace MC, Lindy JD: Chronic stress disorders: Core elements and variations. Final Report to NIMH, Grant No.: R01MH40401-04, 1989a

Green BL, Grace MC, Lindy JD, et al: Comparison of symptom profiles for groups exposed to different traumatic events. Paper presented at the 7th Users Stress Workshop: Training for Psychic Trauma, University of Texas, San Antonio, December 1989b

Green BL, Grace MC, Lindy JD, et al: Risk factors for PTSD and other diagnoses in a general sample of Vietnam veterans. Am J Psychiatry 147:729–733, 1990a

Green BL, Lindy JD, Grace MC, et al: Buffalo Creek survivors in the second decade: Stability of stress symptoms. Am J Orthopsychiatry 60:45–54, 1990b

Helzer JK, Robins LN, McEvoy L; Posttraumatic stress disorder in the general population. New Eng J Med 317:1630–1634, 1987

Kuhne A, Baraga E, Czekala J: Completeness and internal consistency of DSM-III criteria for post-traumatic stress disorder. J Clin Psychol 44:717–722, 1988

Madakasira S, O'Brien KF: Acute post-traumatic stress disorder in victims of a natural disaster. J Nerv Men Dis 175:286–290, 1987

Maida CA, Gordon NS, Steinberg A, et al: Psychosocial impact of disasters: Victims of the Baldwin Hills Fire. Journal of Traumatic Stress 2:37–48, 1989

Myers J, Weissman MM, Tischler GL, et al: Six-month prevalence of psychiatric disorders in three communities. Arch Gen Psychiatry 41:959–967, 1984

North CS, Smith EM, McCool BE, et al: Acute post-disaster coping and adjustment. Journal of Traumatic Stress 2:353–360, 1989

Penk WE, Robinwitz R, Roberts WR, et al: Adjustment differences among male substance abusers, varying in degree of combat experience in Vietnam. J Consult Clin Psychol 49:426–437, 1981

Robins LN, Smith EM: The Diagnostic Interview Schedule Disorder Supplement. St. Louis, MO, Washington University School of Medicine, 1983

Smith EM, North CS: Aftermath of a disaster: Psychological response to the Indianapolis Ramada jet crash. Quick Response Research Report #23. Boulder, CO, Natural Hazards Research and Applications Information Center, 1988

Solomon SD, Canino GJ: Appropriateness of DSM-III-R criteria for post-traumatic stress disorder. Compr Psychiatry 31:227–237, 1990

Steinglass P, Gerrity E: Natural disasters and post-traumatic stress disorder: Short-term versus long-term recovery in two disaster-affected communities. Journal of Applied Social Psychology 20:1746–1765, 1990

Wilkinson CB: Aftermath of a disaster: The collapse of the Hyatt Regency Hotel skywalks. Am J Psychiatry 140:1134–1139, 1983

# ◆ 6 ◆ Symptomatology of Vietnam Veterans With Posttraumatic Stress Disorder

**Terence M. Keane, Ph.D.**

***Summary*** This chapter assesses the adequacy of current criteria for posttraumatic stress disorder (PTSD) in a population of Vietnam combat veterans. To do so, the author focused on reliability of factor structure and internal consistency of the symptoms. The method of clinical evaluation is described, as are the two main dependent measures used. Factors were obtained on both scales that broadly support the conceptualization of PTSD in DSM-III-R (American Psychiatric Association 1987), and good internal cohesiveness was established. These findings are related to other studies and limitations are described, such as choice of population and absence of possibly relevant symptoms.

## Statement of the Issue

The diagnostic criteria for PTSD were introduced into the *Diagnostic and Statistical Manual of Mental Disorders* (DSM-III) in 1980 (American Psychiatric Association 1980). Although the psychological symptoms of traumatic syndromes were included in the DSM-I (American Psychiatric Association 1952) under the rubric of traumatic neuroses, the DSM-II (American Psychiatric Association 1968) omitted such a disorder, preferring to categorize these reactions as transient situational disturbances or gross stress reactions. In the 1960s and 1970s, with the appearance of large numbers of returning Vietnam veterans at public health facilities and veterans medical centers, there was increasing recognition by mental health providers of the symptom constellation that constitutes PTSD as it is now defined. This recognition resulted in the creation of the PTSD diagnostic category for inclusion in the DSM-III. Specifying the criteria was a difficult task for the group of experts assembled for this purpose, because little research existed on the topic of interest. Consequently, the group relied for completion of their task on the many phenomenological and descriptive studies that appeared in the clinical literature describing the aftermath of war, disasters, the Holocaust, and other extreme stressors.

Inclusion of PTSD in the Anxiety Disorders category was consistent with the belief of the majority of experts that a specific stressor was etiologically responsible for the appearance of the disorder and that anxiety was the preeminent symptom associated with a traumatic response. This categorization of PTSD as an anxiety disorder has been somewhat controversial because of the emerging recognition of depression and dissociation as important components of the diagnostic picture of individuals who have been traumatized.

The most recent revision of the DSM, DSM-III-R, essentially agreed that the basic symptoms associated with the disorder should remain relatively intact from one version to the next, although the experts preferred to employ a theoretically driven model for enunciating the PTSD symptoms. Brett and Ostroff (1985) presented a theoretical formulation of PTSD that had its origins in psychoanalytic theory. Positing a bidimensional phenomenology of PTSD that incorporated both intrusive and reliving symptoms, coexisting or alternating with numbing or avoidant symptoms, this model was adopted as the framework for structuring the symptom criteria.

In addition to the use of theory to assist in the specification of DSM criteria, the DSM-III workgroup also examined the available data in order to assist in the process. As a function of numerous published studies regarding the importance of psychophysiological arousal to the PTSD symptomatology (Blanchard et al. 1982; Malloy et al. 1983), a separate set of criteria emphasizing an arousal dimension was included in the revision. Specifically included was a criterion stating that PTSD patients were hyperreactive to cues reminiscent of the trauma as well as numerous signs and symptoms of autonomic arousal (e.g., startle response, sleep disturbance, hypervigilance). In addition, Zimering and colleagues (1984) in directly assessing the presence of the DSM-III criteria for PTSD in patients and controls found that patients with PTSD had a distinct and noticeable deficit in their concentration, while memory per se remained intact. This study resulted in a change in the criteria from memory defects (DSM-III) to concentration impairment (DSM-III-R) as being optimally descriptive of the abnormal process. The DSM-III-R, then, was a result of both theoretical and empirical advances in the study of this disorder.

This combination of factors was a significant improvement upon the atheoretical and unempirical effort undertaken by the original DSM-III group, although clearly theories and data were minimal at the time of their initial work. The preliminary empirical research on PTSD was stimulated by the Veterans Administration in an attempt to help in the readjustment of the millions of soldiers returning from Vietnam and it was this work on combat veterans that supplied much of the data on which the DSM-III-R was based (Blanchard et al. 1982; Egendorf et al. 1981; Keane et al. 1984; Malloy et al. 1983). The theoretical paper by Brett and Ostroff (1985), on which the committee heavily relied, was also a product of research on combat veterans. Although there is greater balance in the literature today, combat and the consequences of war stress remain the topics receiving the greatest attention in the mental health literature on PTSD. For this reason, my discussion in this chapter devotes analytical effort to the data collected on combat veterans with a diagnosis of PTSD.

The issue to be addressed in this chapter is the adequacy of the current diagnostic criteria (DSM-III-R) for combat veterans with PTSD. To examine this issue, data from Vietnam veterans at the Boston PTSD Center are described.

To address the adequacy of the diagnostic criteria for PTSD, I decided to focus on the reliability of the symptomatology, the factor structure of tools constructed to measure PTSD by the DSM-III-R criteria, and the internal consistency of symptom measures in patients who were diagnosed with PTSD. This would provide information on whether the criteria seem to measure a unitary or multiphasic process of psychopathology and if the dimensions identified are strongly related conceptually.

# Method

## Subjects

All subjects evaluated at the Boston PTSD Center and given the PTSD diagnosis according to DSM-III-R criteria were included in this study. Subjects who received a PTSD diagnosis were included in the current study, although this constituted only 77% of the total assessments completed over the 2-year period. Data from a total of 68 patients were analyzed. The mean age of the subjects at the time of assessment was 37 years, and the mean educational level was nearly 13 years. Eighty percent of the subjects were white, and 20% were members of minority groups.

## Diagnostic Measures

To be included in the current study, subjects were evaluated by doctoral-level clinicians in the following manner. Clinicians administered the Jackson Structured Interview for PTSD (Keane et al. 1985) to all subjects. This interview includes demographic information as well as premilitary, military, and postmilitary histories of psychological and social functioning. The Combat Exposure Scale (Keane et al. 1989) provided a subjective estimate of the amount of combat the individual had seen (i.e., trauma exposure). The Minnesota Multiphasic Personality Inventory (MMPI; Hathaway and McKinley 1989) and its PTSD subscale (Keane et al. 1984) and a battery of psychometric scales measuring anxiety (Spielberger State-Trait Anxiety Inventories; Spielberger et al. 1970) and depression (Beck Depression Inventory [BDI]—Beck et al. 1961; Zung 1965) were complemented by the Weissman and Bothwell (1978) Social Adjustment Scale.

To measure PTSD symptoms more directly, the Mississippi Scale for Combat-related PTSD (Keane et al. 1988) was administered; this instrument was keyed to both DSM-III and DSM-III-R criteria and associated features. Next, each subject was given the Structured Clinical Interview for DSM-III-R (SCID; Spitzer and Williams 1985), an interview that covers comprehensively the DSM-III-R criteria for the disorder. For 80% ($n = 54$) of the subjects, a psychophysiological assessment procedure was administered to provide an evaluation of the patients' psychophysiological reactivity to cues symbolic of their combat experience. These results are not presented here.

To arrive at an individual patient's diagnosis, a senior staff meeting was held. This meeting was regularly attended by eight doctoral-level clinical psychologists and the Center's psychiatrist. Presentations incorporated information about the patient's background, history, course of disorder, and presenting symptoms. Data from the psychometrics and the psychophysiological assessment were also included in the presentation. Case formulation, diagnostic considerations, and treatment recommendations composed the objectives for each patient. Axis I and Axis II diagnoses were conferred when appropriate. If all diagnostic indicators were in agreement, consensus diagnosis was readily achieved. In those cases where the indicators disagreed, the team would discuss the case to arrive at the diagnoses that were deemed most appropriate by consensus.

## Evaluation of Instrumentation

For purposes of this project, the instruments to be examined were those instruments most closely aligned with the DSM-III-R criteria. The SCID having been developed directly from the DSM-III-R criteria and the Mississippi Scale having been keyed to the DSM-III and DSM-III-R, these two instruments were the ones selected for evaluation. It was hypothesized that the diagnostic criteria were appropriate if the psychometric properties of these two instruments were strong.

To assess the psychometric properties of these instruments the following analyses were conducted: 1) Cronbach's alpha coefficient, 2) item–total score mean correlation, and 3) a principal components analysis. In addition, the mean ratings for the Mississippi Scale items were examined to determine the relative frequency for which the items that represent DSM-III-R criteria were endorsed by PTSD patients.

# Results

## Structured Clinical Interview for DSM-III-R

A principal components analysis was conducted on the 15 variables that compose the B through D symptoms of the PTSD diagnosis. Table 6–1 presents information on the items loading on each factor. Factors were identified as those with eigenvalues greater than 1.0 following a varimax rotation. Inspection of a scree plot yielded an array of four factors that most adequately described the variables examined. An item had to load at .50 to be considered part of a characterized factor. For the SCID, factor 1 describes intrusive experiences, reliving experiences, restriction of affect, and hypervigilance. Factor 2 includes items pertaining to reactivity,

| Table 6–1. | Items composing each factor of the principal components analysis of the Structural Clinical Interview for DSM-III-R |
|---|---|

**Factor 1**
1. Recurrent nightmares of the event
2. Sudden acting or feeling as if the vent were recurring
3. Restricted range of affect
4. Hypervigilance

**Factor 2**
1. Physiological reactivity or intense distress at exposure to events that resemble the trauma

2. Deliberate effects to avoid activities or situations that resemble the trauma
3. Exaggerated startle responses

**Factor 3**
1. Irritability or outbursts of anger
2. Concentration difficulties

**Factor 4**
1. Markedly diminished interest in significant activities
2. Feelings of detachment or estrangement

avoidance, and startle. Included in factor 3 are two Criterion D stimuli, irritability and concentration impairment. Factor 4 includes two items from Criterion C in that it contains a markedly diminished interest in activities and also feelings of detachment or estrangement. These factors are generally supportive of the conceptual model that drove the DSM-III-R in that reliving, avoidance, and arousal symptoms seemed to cluster together for PTSD patients. This was true irrespective of the range of possible scores (1 to 3) for each symptom and the relatively small number of subjects (68). The restricted range of affect loaded on the same factor as reliving items and as such might be considered a part of (or a function of) the intrusive memories of trauma.

Cronbach's alpha coefficient was calculated to be .93 for all 15 symptoms assessed by the SCID, indicating a high propensity for the DSM-III-R criteria to operate interdependently. It is also an indication of high reliability of items across the many subjects. In many respects the items appear to measure a unitary dimension of disorder across all symptom areas.

Item–total score correlations averaged .70 with a range of scores extending from .54 to .85. This indicates that for subjects each item on the SCID rating scale is related in an acceptable way to the overall score provided by summing scores on all symptoms.

## Mississippi Scale for Combat-Related PTSD

The principal components analysis for the Mississippi Scale was conducted on the 35 items of the scale. The same method of analysis was applied here as for the SCID analysis with factors extracted with eigenvalues greater than one. A varimax rotation was employed. Items were considered part of a factor if they loaded with a score of .50 or greater. Examination of a scree plot yielded a four factor solution as optimal. Table 6–2 presents information on the items included in each of the factors.

Factor 1 includes 9 items that clearly reflect reexperiencing phenomena, daydreams, nightmares, and other forms of reliving of the traumatic event. It supports the position of including as reexperiencing those symptoms that represent distress at exposure to events symbolic of the trauma. Factor 2 included a preponderance of items reflecting numbing and restriction of affect with a concomitant use of anger and irritability to dispel these numb feelings.

Factor 3 centers on problems with impulse control or problems in acting out destructive impulses, while factor 4 includes items that reflect on inability to concentrate on or enjoy activities or people in one's life.

Thus, these factors represent the symptom picture of reliving experiences, numbing of affect, impulse control deficits, and cognitive and emotional effectiveness. Their overlap with the DSM-III-R criteria is acceptable although not exact. Many of the arousal symptoms are seen as associated with the reliving, intrusive recollections of the traumatic event. This factor structure is certainly a reasonable framework for viewing the consequences of traumatic experiences.

Cronbach's alpha coefficient was found to be .89 indicating excellent in-

---

**Table 6–2.**    Items composing the four factors of the Mississippi Scale derived from the principal components analysis

---

**Factor 1**

1. Distress at exposure to events reminiscent of the trauma
2. Nightmares
3. Intrusive thoughts
4. Survivor guilt
5. Reliving experiences
6. Daydreams
7. Alienation/detachment

**Factor 2**

1. Numbing/avoidance
2. Restricted affect

3. Irritability and anger
4. Arousal, vigilance
5. Expression of feelings difficult

**Factor 3**

1. Violence and aggression
2. Suicide
3. Frightening urges

**Factor 4**

1. Diminished interest in significant activities
2. Concentration impairment
3. Alienation/estrangement from others

---

ternal stability of the items comprising the Mississippi Scale and again potentially indicating a unified dimension of psychopathology subsumed by the many items included in the scale. The mean item–total score correlation was found to be .47, indicating an acceptable range of the contribution of individual items to the overall performance of the scale.

Examination of subjects' performance on individual items of the Mississippi Scale was accomplished in two ways: those items with the highest endorsements of subjects on average and those items with the lowest mean endorsements by subjects. Table 6–3 contains those items that received an average greater than 4 on the 5-point Likert Scale as well as those items that received a mean lower than 3 on the 5-point scale.

# Discussion

The psychometric analyses on the PTSD criteria from the SCID and the items on the Mississippi Scale provide reasonable support for the current classification scheme. Highlights of the clustering of items suggest that reliving/intrusive phenomena, restricted emotions and numbing, physical reactivity and concomitant avoidance, and diminished interest in activities and in other people are relatively independent factors and compose different dimensions of the disorder. This closely resembles what was intended by the DSM-III-R committee.

The finding that each of the two scales of PTSD, one clinician rated and the other patient self-administered, yielded somewhat similar dimensions of the disorder provides support for the multidimensional notion of the disorder. The high coefficient alphas for each of the scales indicates that the items do seem to be reliably measuring a unitary concept such as PTSD,

---

**Table 6–3.**   Items on the Mississippi Scale that are most strongly endorsed and least strongly endorsed by PTSD subjects

| Items with an average > 4.0 | | |
|---|---|---|
| 1. Detachment/estrangement from others | 6. | Vocational, interpersonal detachment |
| 2. Anger and aggression control | 7. | Startle response |
| 3. Distress at exposure to events that symbolize the trauma | 8. | Alcohol/drug use |
| | 9. | Hypervigilance |
| 4. Sleep disturbance | **Items with an average < 3.0** | |
| 5. Survivor guilt | 1. | Suicide |
| | 2. | Depression (crying spells) |

despite the presence of multiple dimensions or factors. The moderate to high scores on the individual item–total score analyses supports the relative contributions of the items to the overall diagnostic scores. This supports continued inclusion of these items in our attempts to measure the PTSD construct.

The items on the Mississippi Scale that were least frequently endorsed by PTSD patients consisted of suicide and the presence of crying spells. There may be value in maintaining the suicide item as a low-frequency but highly important assessment question. The questions regarding crying spells and suicide may also help discriminate PTSD with its many depressive features from a major depression. This distinction has been discussed in many conceptual articles and also in empirical studies and should continue to be an important arena for research. Because neither symptom is considered a criterion for the disorder, criterion change is not necessary as a result of these findings.

In conclusion, the current study employed well-defined patients with combat-related PTSD. Their responses to questions regarding the DSM-III-R diagnostic criteria for PTSD demonstrate that the symptomatology does indeed capture much of their psychological and interpersonal experiences. These data do not, however, provide firm support for the idea that these are the only symptoms that might be related to PTSD. Nor do they provide support for the notion that these symptoms discriminate PTSD from other psychological disorders in the most parsimonious way.

# Conclusion

The results of this project provide support for the findings of other studies that used combat veterans as subjects. Silver and Iaconno (1984) factor analyzed a scale that was locally developed to assess the symptoms of undiagnosed combat veterans. Their findings were similar in that they found factors of reliving/intrusiveness, depression, anger and irritability, and interpersonal detachment. They advocated the inclusion of depression and anger as central components of PTSD. Although they were correct in their indications that PTSD incorporates depressive symptomatology, anger, irritability, and often rage, it seems likely that these symptoms, though frequently present among PTSD patients, may not provide any incremental discriminability of PTSD from other disorders such as affective disorders, antisocial personality disorder, other personality disorders, and adjustment disorders.

In a similar study, Watson and colleagues (1991) developed a PTSD Inventory, administered it to 131 Vietnam veterans, and factor analyzed it to determine how symptoms clustered together for those patients who reached the criteria for PTSD. In this study, a PTSD diagnosis was dependent exclusively on patients' scores on this instrument. The interview composed items taken directly from the DSM-III criterion for PTSD. The results of the study indicated support for Brett and Ostroff's conceptualization of PTSD (1985), arriving at five factors to describe the interrelated dimensions of disorder. The greatest point of overlap with the current study was in the strong relationship of traumalike stimuli worsening symptoms overlapping with intrusive thoughts and reliving experiences. Both my discussion here and the study of Watson and colleagues would posit a reconsideration of the placement of that particular criterion. The original validational study of the Mississippi Scale also supports this specific finding (Keane et al. 1988).

Watson and colleagues (1991) also found strong support for a separate dimension for detachment, constricted affect, and numbing to intimacy (Factor 3). These results bolster the inclusion of these symptoms as a potentially separate dimension among combat veterans.

## Concerns About the Process Involved in Statistical Approaches to Diagnosis

Considerable attention was given to the possible use of the National Vietnam Veterans Readjustment Study (NVVRS; Kulka et al. 1990) data set to help in the process described here. Many issues arose in the discussions with the NVVRS investigators that prompted us not to use that data set because of the expense involved and our inability to unravel some crucial issues. Our concerns may be useful to the group as a whole and can be summarized as follows:

1. To properly evaluate what symptoms are associated with PTSD, the whole domain of possible symptoms should be sampled so that important ones are not unintentionally overlooked. Unfortunately, in the Boston PTSD Center and in the NVVRS, the clear focus was on sampling symptoms thought to be associated with PTSD on an a priori basis. This

limitation affects our capacity to be sure we have evaluated all possible symptoms that might serve as criteria.

2. The population in the NVVRS was non-help-seeking, and it was unclear to all involved that symptoms expressed by this group of individuals would be representative of those who are help-seeking. Does seeking help have a role to play in determining disorder? Does current social, vocational, interpersonal functioning play a role in determining disorder?

3. The question of who has the disorder was intensely discussed. There is considerable circularity in the notion that those people who should be studied are those that have the disorder, because this presumes that the current criteria are accurate (valid) and can serve to guide us in a statistical or otherwise meaningful way. For example, should patients or subjects not be studied if they meet DSM-III-R Criteria A, B, D, and E, but do not meet the numbing criterion, C? This problem of circularity creates considerable confusion when trying to arrive at any sensible method for studying PTSD.

4. The problem of considering PTSD as a continuous variable versus a dichotomous one is a related concern. Many would state that the disorder is either present or absent, when it is most reasonable from our instrumentation to consider PTSD as a continuous variable. Yet the DSM calls for artificially considering PTSD (and most other disorders) as a dichotomy. To arrive at such trenchant distinctions among the disorders and among symptom criteria is probably premature given the available technology for measurement.

With so many of the patients with PTSD also meeting criteria for other disorders (Keane and Wolfe 1990) it is unclear which symptoms are central to PTSD and which ones are secondary to the presence of other disorders. This problem is especially difficult, because lifetime substance abuse is associated with PTSD in 60–80% of the cases.

In summary, the presence of these problems renders many data sets unusable for the purpose of studying diagnostic criteria. Major data sets are frequently constructed surrounding extant diagnostic criteria. This problem renders these sets inadequate for purposes of elucidating diagnostic criteria, because bias has already been introduced by the choice of measures. The difficulty of who to study is also an important issue. If only patients who meet diagnostic criteria are included in these studies, then the bias in favor of preexisting criteria is obvious. Should we decide to open the gates to a broader subject population, then we are, de facto, considering the disorder as a continuous variable. This would not be satisfactory to many investigators or clinicians.

Finally, it is important to consider what defines disorder and also what symptoms should be included in the criteria. Is disorder help-seeking? This is certainly inadequate. Is disorder functional impairment (vocational or otherwise)? This also presents a morass for investigators.

Although the approach taken in this chapter has been a statistical one, it has some serious limitations that need to be stated forthrightly. Subject selection, sampling of the measures of the construct, the debate over what should be included in diagnostic criteria, and the discussion of how we should define disorder all contribute to ambivalence in making any strong recommendations for changing the diagnostic criteria for PTSD at this time.

# References

American Psychiatric Association: Diagnostic and Statistical Manual: Mental Disorders. Washington, DC, American Psychiatric Association, 1952

American Psychiatric Association: Diagnostic and Statistical Manual of Mental Disorders, 2nd Edition. Washington, DC, American Psychiatric Association, 1968

American Psychiatric Association: Diagnostic and Statistical Manual of Mental Disorders, 3rd Edition. Washington, DC, American Psychiatric Association, 1980

American Psychiatric Association: Diagnostic and Statistical Manual of Mental Disorders, 3rd Edition, Revised. Washington, DC, American Psychiatric Association, 1987

Beck AT, Ward CH, Mendelson M, et al: An inventory for measuring depression. Arch Gen Psychiatry 12:63–70, 1961

Blanchard EB, Kolb LC, Pallmeyer TB, et al: The development of a psychophysiological assessment procedure for post-traumatic stress disorder in Vietnam veterans. Psychiatr Q 54:220–229, 1982

Brett EA, Ostroff R: Imagery and posttraumatic stress disorder: an overview. Am J Psychiatry 142:417–424, 1985

Egendorf A, Kadushin C, Laufer RS, et al (eds): Legacies of Vietnam: Comparative Adjustment of Veterans and Their Peers, Vol V. New York, Center for Policy Research, 1981

Hathaway SR, McKinley JC: Minnesota Multiphasic Personality Inventory—2. Minneapolis, MN, University of Minnesota, 1989

Keane TM, Wolfe J: Comorbidity in post-traumatic stress disorder: an analysis of community and clinical studies. Journal of Applied Social Psychology 20:1776–1788, 1990

Keane TM, Malloy PF, Fairbank JA: Empirical development of an MMPI subscale for the assessment of combat-related posttraumatic stress disorder. J Consult Clin Psychol 52:888–891, 1984

Keane TM, Fairbank JA, Caddell JM, et al: A behavioral approach to assessing and treating posttraumatic stress disorder in Vietnam veterans, in Trauma and Its Wake. Edited by Figley CR. New York, Brunner/Mazel, 1985, pp 257–294

Keane TM, Caddell JM, Taylor KL: Mississippi scale for combat-related posttraumatic stress disorder: three studies in reliability and validity. J Consult Clin Psychol 56:85–90, 1988

Keane TM, Fairbank JA, Caddell JM, et al: Clinical evaluation of a measure to assess combat exposure. Psychological Assessment: A Journal of Consulting and Clinical Psychology 1:53–55, 1989

Kulka RA, Schlenger WE, Fairbank JA, et al: Trauma and the Vietnam War Generation. New York, Brunner/Mazel, 1990

Malloy PF, Fairbank JA, Keane TM: Validation of a multimethod assessment of posttraumatic stress disorders in Vietnam veterans. J Consult Clin Psychol 51:488–494, 1983

Silver SM, Iacono CU: Factor-analytic support for DSM-III's post-traumatic stress disorder for Vietnam veterans. J Clin Psychol 40:5–14, 1984

Spielberger CB, Goresuch RL, Lushene RE: Manual for the State-Trait Inventory (self-evaluation questionnaire). Palo Alto, CA, Consulting Psychologists Press, 1970

Spitzer R, Williams J: Structured clinical interview for DSM-III (SCID). New York, Biometrics Research Department of New York State Psychiatric Institute, 1985

Watson CG, Kucala T, Juba M, et al: A factor analysis of the DSM-III Post-traumatic Stress Disorder criteria. J Clin Psychol 47:205–214, 1991

Weissman MM, Bothwell S: Assessment of social adjustment by patient self report. Arch Gen Psychiatry 33:1111–1115, 1976

Zimering RT, Caddell JM, Fairbank JA, et al: PTSD in Vietnam veterans: an empirical evaluation of the diagnostic criteria. Paper presented at the annual meeting of the Association for the Advancement of Behavior Therapy, Philadelphia, PA, November 1984

Zung WWK: A self-rating depression scale. Arch Gen Psychiatry 12:63–70, 1965

# ◆ 7 ◆ Posttraumatic Stress Disorder Associated With Exposure to Criminal Victimization in Clinical and Community Populations

Dean G. Kilpatrick, Ph.D.
Heidi S. Resnick, Ph.D.

**Summary**  **B**ased on a literature review of criminal victimization, as well as on their work, the authors make suggestions on six aspects of posttraumatic stress disorder (PTSD): 1) specificity of symptoms to trauma; 2) prevalence of exposure to criminal victimization in the community; 3) rates of crime induced PTSD across different populations, with varied criteria based on duration of symptoms; 4) effects of crime type and feature upon prevalence of PTSD; 5) psychiatric comorbidity; and 6) frequency of individual symptoms and patterns of co-occurrence. Study samples are described, along with results relevant to the above issues. The authors bring the results of their survey to bear on further refining the criteria for PTSD, on its descriptive characterization, and outline a method for studying many of the questions raised both by themselves and by authors of other chapters in this book.

## Statement of the Issue

This chapter provides a comprehensive review of the literature relevant to the text of DSM-IV; it also provides an examination of data available re-

113

garding patterns of individual symptoms of PTSD. Topics addressed include the following:

1. Methodological issues, including decision rules regarding specificity of symptom items to specific trauma experienced;
2. Prevalence of exposure to various types of criminal victimization within community samples;
3. Rates of PTSD across a variety of sample populations, with varied criteria for duration of symptoms, as well as rates of current PTSD at different time periods postcrime;
4. Differential rates of PTSD associated with various crime types as well as within crime characteristics;
5. PTSD comorbidity with other diagnoses; and
6. Frequency and rank order of individual symptoms across sample types, as well as patterns of co-occurrence of symptoms.

# Results

## Methodological Issues

Study samples are described in Table 7–1, and features of the 11 studies are included in Table 7–2. It is these numbers that are used in the text. It is apparent that there was wide variation in methodological characteristics, including diagnostic decision rules, settings, and sampled populations. The most frequently used PTSD assessment interview was the Diagnostic Interview Schedule (DIS) or some modified version of the DIS (used in 5 studies). However, even within this set of studies, there was variation in terms of whether symptom items were required to be linked with a specific stressor on the part of the subject.

For example, in all but one of the studies we included from our own research with community samples, only one reexperiencing item had to be specifically linked to the trauma as a criterion for diagnosis, whereas in sample 6 and sample 2 methods, all items had to be linked with the trauma. The majority of samples were specially referred by community agencies or crisis centers. In almost half of the samples, those restricted to direct victims of sexual assault or rape, included only female victims. A wide variety of crime trauma categories were included, ranging from indirect victimization associated with homicide, assault, or rape of a family member to direct exposure to criminal assault and sniper attack, with rape being the most frequent type of direct victimization experience. Finally, the time since assault at which subjects were assessed ranged from approximately 2 weeks postassault to

---

Table 7–1.   Sample identification table

| Study/Sample | Reference Number |
|---|---|
| Foa and Rothbaum, unpublished, 1989—The impact of rape on dyadic involvement and functioning; NIMH Grant Number: MH29602 . . . . . . . . . . . . | 1 |
| Rothbaum et al. 1988—Responses following sexual and nonsexual assault . . . . . . . . . . . . . . . . . . . . . . . . | 1a |
| Kilpatrick et al. 1987b—The psychological impact of crime; NIJ Grant Number: 84-IJ-CX-0039 . . . . . . . . . . . . . . . . . . . . . . . . . | 2 |
| Kilpatrick et al. 1989b—Victim and crime factors associated with the development of crime-related posttraumatic stress disorder . . . . . . . . . . | 2a |
| Kilpatrick et al. 1987a—Criminal victimization: Lifetime prevalence, reporting to police, and psychological impact . . . . . . . . . . . . . . . . . . | 2b |
| Veronen and Saunders 1989—Rape relationship project; NIMH Grant Number: MH40360 . . . . . . . . . . . . . . . . . . . . . . . . . . | 3 |
| Resnick et al. 1988—Symptoms of PTSD in rape victims and their partners . . . . | 3a |
| Resnick et al., unpublished, 1989—Preliminary data analyses: Assessment of PTSD in a subset of rape victims at 12 to 36 months postassault . . . . . . . . . | 3b |
| Kilpatrick et al. 1989a—Victims rights and services in South Carolina; JAA Grant Number: 86-024 . . . . . . . . . . . . . . . . . . . . . . . . . . . . . | 4 |
| Kilpatrick et al. 1989a—Preliminary data analyses direct victims . . . . . . . . . . . . | 4a |
| Kilpatrick et al. 1989a—Preliminary data analyses family members . . . . . . . . . . | 4b |
| Kilpatrick et al. 1990—The impact of homicide on surviving family members; NIJ Grant Number: 87-IJ-CX-0017 . . . . . . . . . . . . . . . . . . . . . . . | 5 |
| Amick et al. 1989—Public health implications of homicide for surviving family members . . . . . . . . . . . . . . . . . . . . . . . . . | 5a |
| Kilpatrick et al. 1989c—Family members of homicide victims: Search for meaning and posttraumatic stress disorder . . . . . . . . . . . . . . . | 5b |
| Helzer et al. 1987—posttraumatic stress disorder in the general population findings of the epidemiologic catchment area survey . . . . . . . . . . | 6 |
| Frank and Anderson 1987—Psychiatric disorders in rape victims: Past history and current symptomatology . . . . . . . . . . . . . . . . . . . . . . . | 7 |
| McLeer et al. 1988—posttraumatic stress disorder in sexually abused children . . . . . . | 8 |
| Pynoos and Nader 1988—Children who witness the sexual assaults of their mothers . . . . . . . . . . . . . . . . . . . . . . . . . . . . . . . . . . . | 9 |
| Pynoos et al. 1987—Life threat and posttraumatic stress in school-age children . . . . | 10 |
| Kilpatrick et al. 1989d— Risk factors for substance abuse; NIDA Grant Number: DA 05220 . . . . . . . . . . | 11 |
| Kilpatrick 1990—Violence as a precursor of women's substance abuse: The rest of the drugs-violence story . . . . . . . . . . . . . . . . . . . . . . . . . . . | 11a |

**Table 7–2.** Sample tables—PTSD symptomatology or diagnoses in victims of crime (design features)

| Study reference number | Number | Method | Setting | Groups | Percent Male | Age | Percent White | Time Since Crime |
|---|---|---|---|---|---|---|---|---|
| 1 | 61 rape victims 51 crime victims[a] | Structured interview for PTSD DSM-III criteria | Referral community agencies Philadelphia | Rape/ crime | Crime only 39.2% | Median 25/36 | 38.4 | Weekly longitudinal assessment[b] |

[a]From 1a report based on 57 rape/37 crime. Crimes included robbery, simple or aggravated assault. Assessment at 1, 4, 6, 8, 12 weeks, 3 months, 6 months, and 1 year.
[b]One week is initial assessment, not necessarily 1 week postrape for all subjects.

| Study reference number | Number | Method | Setting | Groups | Percent Male | Age | Percent White | Time Since Crime |
|---|---|---|---|---|---|---|---|---|
| 2 | 295 crime 96 control 391 total 41.9% of target population | Structured interview for DSM-III PTSD SCID-type[a] | Community sample from larger random sample Charleston | Completed & attemped rape; sexual assault; physical assault; robbery; burglary | 0 | Mean 39.8 | 72.9 | 15 years |

[a]PTSD Assessment: Trauma assessed separately from assessment of symptoms, then questions asked in specific reference to single or worst crime. The interview items used phrasing similar to the structured clinical interview for DSM-III-R (SCID). Also, like the SCID there were no item skips in the PTSD interview schedule.

| Study reference number | Number | Method | Setting | Groups | Percent Male | Age | Percent White | Time Since Crime |
|---|---|---|---|---|---|---|---|---|
| 3 | 108 rape victim 84 control victims 9 rape partners: 38 rape 42 control[a] | SCID interview on 33 victims 9 rape partners DSM-III-R[b] | Referral crisis center Matched controls Charleston | Rape/ control | 29.4% | 28.84 F 29.54 M | 64.1 F | 2 weeks longitudinal |

[a]Demographic data based on preliminary descriptives of subjects who completed any portion of protocol.
[b]SCID modified so that items were asked in specific reference to recent rape, only a subset of the larger sample who returned for assessment at 12–36 months were administered the SCID. Other assessment periods included self-report measures only.

| 4 | 128 direct & 123 family members Crime victims 251 total | Structured interview DSM-III-R PTSD phone modified DIS[a] | ID'd by CJS contact South Carolina | Homicide; aggravated assault; sexual assault; robbery; burglary | 36.7 | 38.2 | 62.5 | Mode: ≤ 2 years |
|---|---|---|---|---|---|---|---|---|
| 5 | 214 close family members criminal- & alcohol-related vehicular homicide | Structured interview DSM-III-R phone modified DIS[a] | Random sample national | Criminal vehicular homicide | 31.3 | 43.5 | 66.1 control 82.4 victim | 16.62 years |
| 6 | 2,493 67% of target population | Structured interview DIS DSM-III PTSD | ECA St. Louis oversampling of blacks | Combat; accident; physical assault; seeing violence; threat; natural disaster; other | 38.7[a] | | | Not specified[b] |

[a]DIS modification: Only reexperiencing criterion items were required to be specific to identified victimization; symptoms of avoidance of thoughts/feelings, places/activities asked in reference to "something that had happened in the past"; all other symptoms (i.e., sleep, concentration, decreased interest, etc.) were not asked in reference to past event, either general or specific to victimization included all DSM-III-R symptom items, except psychogenic amnesia, worsening of mood to reminders, changed view of future.

[a]DIS modification: Only reexperiencing criterion items were required to be specific to identified victimization; symptoms of avoidance of thoughts/feelings, places/activities asked in reference to "something that had happened in the past"; all other symptoms (i.e., sleep, concentration, decreased interest, etc.) were not asked in reference to past event, either general or specific to victimization. All DSM-III-R symptom items, except psychogenic amnesia, worsening of mood to reminders, changed view of future.

[a]All combat cases were male, from Vietnam combat.
[b]Three assessments: initial and 2 follow-ups at 6 months each; time since trauma not specified except for mugging which was past 18 months.

Table 7–2.  Sample tables—PTSD symptomatology or diagnoses in victims of crime (design features)  (continued)

| Study reference number | Number | Method | Setting | Groups | Percent Male | Age | Percent White | Time Since Crime |
|---|---|---|---|---|---|---|---|---|
| 7 | 60 rape 31 control | Mod DIS structured DSM-III PTSD interview[a] structured interview | Crisis center referrals Pittsburgh | Rape control | 0 | — | 23.4 | Longitudinal[b] |

[a]12 of 60 rape victims were assessed for PTSD at end of study, because the PTSD section was included in the interview after the remaining subjects had completed the protocol.
[b]Subjects were assessed initially, postrape, after 14 weeks and 6 months.

| Study reference number | Number | Method | Setting | Groups | Percent Male | Age | Percent White | Time Since Crime |
|---|---|---|---|---|---|---|---|---|
| 8 | 31 | Structured interview DSM-III-R | Child outpatient psychiatry | Sexual abuse | 19.35 | — | 8.4 | 8 months |
| 9 | 10 | PTSD reaction index DSM-III interview | Referral crisis mental health | Witness mother sexual assault[a] | 70.0 | 15–17 | Predominately white | — |

[a]Not clear whether all assaults were completed rapes.

| Study reference number | Number | Method | Setting | Groups | Percent Male | Age | Percent White | Time Since Crime |
|---|---|---|---|---|---|---|---|---|
| 10 | 159 | Child PTSD reaction index DSM-III interview | 14.5% of student body at elementary school | Sniper attack on playground | 50.3 | 50% Black 50% Hispanic | 9.2 | 1 month |
| 11 | 1,549 1,101 (71.1%) trauma victims 48 nonvictims | Structured interview DSM-III-R phone modified DIS[a] | National Random sample | Crime other trauma | 0 | 35–39 victim mode 40–44 nonvictim | 86% | 9.7–24 years preliminary estimate |

[a]DIS modification: Only reexperiencing criterion items were required to be specific to identified victimization; symptoms of avoidance of thoughts/feelings, places/activities, worsening of mood to reminders, physiological reactivity to reminders, changed view of future, and psychogenic amnesia asked in reference to "something that had happened in the past"; all other symptoms (i.e., sleep, concentration, decreased interest, etc.) were not asked in reference to past event, either general or specific to victimization.

approximately 17 years. Only one study (Study #1) assessed symptoms longitudinally using a structured interview. Based on the variety of design features of the studies, ability to compare findings across samples is limited, and results of comparisons must be interpreted with caution.

## Exposure Rates

Criterion A as currently defined in DSM-III-R (American Psychiatric Association 1987) is described as an "event that is outside the range of usual human experience and that would be markedly distressing to almost anyone" (p. 247). Examples of this type of event include criminal victimization such as physical assault, including rape, as well as serious harm to a family member or close friend. A central question is whether or not more common events should be included in Criterion A, or even whether this criterion should be kept at all as the rate-limiting step required for a diagnosis of PTSD. Regardless of whether Criterion A is broadened or eliminated from the diagnostic category and routinely assessed in the category of current stressors, information about the prevalence of exposure to various types of events that may produce high rates of symptomatology is important. In addition, the development of assessment measures that are valid and reliable measures of exposure to potentially traumatic events is crucial, whether criminal victimization or a broader category of stressors is being measured.

With respect to exposure to criminal victimization, data from four community samples included in Table 7–3 indicate that many crimes are neither rare events nor outside the realm of normal human experience. In the victimization research area, methodological factors such as use of sensitive and comprehensive screening instruments detect higher rates of criminal victimization experiences than those obtained with government crime surveys, which use broad questions about crimes in general (and rape in particular). The methodology employed in our own samples included assessment of up to three criminal victimizations per respondent: the first, the most recent, and the worst. Crimes were defined using specific behavioral descriptions that allowed for identification of events (such as assaults by a family member) that would not otherwise have been labeled as crimes by the subject. With regard to direct victimization, the findings indicate that a history of completed rape was reported by between 13% and 23% of adult women, whereas rates for any type of sexual assault ranged from 24% to 53%. The rates observed for physical or aggravated assault ranged from 2.8% within the past 18 months alone to 11.1% for lifetime occurrence.

With respect to secondary victimization, total criminal and vehicular homicide deaths of family members or friends totalled 9.3% in one national sample of adult men and woman (Study #5a), and 14.3% in a second sample of women only (Study #11).

Results from Study #11 indicate that a large portion of the total sample (33.6%; this subgroup was noncrime) reported other types of potentially traumatic events aside from criminal victimization. These data are preliminary, and further analyses of subjects' identified traumatic events and objective responses to assessment of life stress and associated distress will be

**Table 7–3.** Prevalence of exposure to criminal victimization in community samples (percentages)

| Type of Crime/Event | 2a | 5a | 6 | 11 |
|---|---|---|---|---|
| Completed rape | 23.3 | | | 12.9 |
| Attempted rape | 13.1 | | | |
| Completed molestation | 18.4 | | | 3.0 |
| Attempted molestation | 4.6 | | | |
| Attempted sexual assault, general | | | | 8.0 |
| Other sexual assault | 3.9 | | | |
| Total sexual assault | 53.0 | | | 24.0 |
| Aggravated assault | 9.7 | | 2.77[a] | 11.1 |
| Robbery | 5.6 | | | |
| Burglary | 45.3 | | | |
| Criminal homicide | 3.8 | | | 9.7 |
| Vehicular homicide | 5.4 | | | 4.6 |
| Total other trauma[b] | | | 33.6 | |
|     Natural disaster | | | | 14.1 |
|     Witness injury or death | | | | 10.1 |
|     Serious injury or physical damage | | | | 3.4 |
|     Feared death or serious injury | | | | 4.4 |
|     Serious accident | | | | 10.7 |
|     Other extraordinary stressful event | | | | 14.3 |
| Vietnam combat | | | 1.72 | |
| Wounded in combat | | | .60 | |
| Total crime/event | 75.4 | 9.3 | | 71.1 |

[a] This rate in study 6 is for past 18 months only.
[b] These rates were obtained for women who had never been crime victims, and subcategories *are not* mutually exclusive.

relevant to the issue of broadening Criterion A, or reassigning the assessment of a stressor to Axis IV.

Another issue relates to the assessment of PTSD when a person has been exposed to a variety of traumatic events. Data from Study #2a indicated that 75% of the women interviewed had been victims of at least one crime. Additionally, of that group of 295 women, only 85 reported just one victimization. In the assessment of PTSD, respondents were required to report symptoms in reference to the only or worst crime they had experienced. In Study #11, in addition to the 33.6% of the sample that reported other trauma only, 28.7% of the crime victims also reported having experienced "other" trauma. Clearly this makes the assessment of PTSD specific to an event a complicated matter. There are no guidelines at present to help clarify this issue. The suggestions proposed by Solomon and Canino (1990) and the position advocated by Green (1990)—to first assess Criterion B, C, and D symptoms and then work backward to an assessment of trauma exposure, and in this case multiple trauma history—might be the optimal method of empirically evaluating the association between this pattern of distress and a variety of events and event patterns.

Because Study #11 collected information about the lifetime prevalence of a variety of potentially traumatic events and about lifetime and current PTSD prevalence, it provides an opportunity to examine the issue of which types of potentially traumatic events are most prevalent among the life histories of those women who developed PTSD and among those who had PTSD currently at the time of assessment. As Table 7–4 indicates, certain potentially traumatic events appeared to be more prevalent in the life histories of the lifetime PTSD positive group than the lifetime base rate for that event within the entire sample. For example, 12.9% of the sample had experienced completed rape, and 11.1% had a history of aggravated assault. However, 33% of those with lifetime PTSD had a history of rape, and 32% had a history of aggravated assault. In contrast, the lifetime prevalence for "other" traumatic events only (33.6%) was higher than the probability that those in the lifetime PTSD group would have a history of "other" traumatic events only (25%).

With respect to current PTSD, 49% of those with current PTSD had a history of rape and 41% had a history of aggravated assault. Only 14% of those with current PTSD had histories of traumatic events other than crime. This indicates that a history of completed rape or aggravated assault

Table 7–4.  Base rates for potentially traumatic events, lifetime and current PTSD, and traumatic event probabilities within lifetime and current PTSD groups from national probability sample of 1,539 adult women

| Potential Traumatic Event | Lifetime Event Prevalence (%) | Lifetime PTSD Prevalence (%) | Event Probability Within Lifetime PTSD Group (%) | Current PTSD Prevalence (%) | Event Probability Within Current PTSD Group (%) |
|---|---|---|---|---|---|
| Completed rape | 12.9 | 35 | 33 | 13 | 49 |
| Sexual molestation | 3.0 | 23 | 5 | 2 | 1 |
| Attempted sexual assault | 8.0 | 23 | 14 | 7 | 18 |
| Aggravated assault | 11.1 | 39 | 32 | 12 | 41 |
| Homicide death of family or friend | 9.7 | 24 | 17 | 7 | 20 |
| Drunk driving death of family or friend | 4.6 | 27 | 9 | 4 | 6 |
| Other traumatic event only | 33.6 | 10 | 25 | 1 | 14 |

appears to place women at higher risk for PTSD development and maintenance than the prevalence of these events themselves would suggest.

## PTSD Rates and Time Since Trauma

Overall rates of lifetime and/or current PTSD observed in the 11 samples are included in Table 7–5. An observation of the varying criteria for duration of symptoms employed across studies raises another question related to diagnostic decision rules. To our knowledge, no empirical basis exists for the requirement of 1 month duration of symptoms included in DSM-III-R rules. This issue is addressed elsewhere in this volume (see Chapter 1 by Blank and Chapter 2 by Rothbaum and Foa) and will not be addressed in detail here. However, this important methodological difference must be taken into account when comparing observed PTSD rates across studies. In Study #1, the initial assessment was not necessarily conducted immediately postcrime, but was the earliest assessment. Similarly, the 4-week assessment of current PTSD can be viewed as indicating symptomatology that was present for at least 4 weeks and may be a conservative estimate. These results indicate a substantial reduction in PTSD rates at the two assessments.

Similarly, the rates observed in rape victims in Study #3b, in which subjects 12–36 months postrape retrospectively reported whether they ever had a symptom and whether the problem lasted for at least 1 month or more, were greatly reduced when the 1-month criterion was applied. An examination of lifetime rates of PTSD in the three samples with data where a 1-month criterion may be applied (Studies #1, #3a/3b, and #11) indicated a range of from 19% in a general crime and other trauma national probability sample (Study #11) to rates of between 51% and 61% in two community/crisis agency referred samples. In general, rates of lifetime PTSD without the 1-month criterion ranged from lows of 23.4% in a national probability homicide survivor sample (Study #5a) and 27.8% in a community general crime group (Study #2b), to higher rates ranging from approx-

**Table 7–5.**   PTSD rates in the 11 study samples

| Study | Duration/Recency Criteria | Lifetime (%) | Time Since | Current (%) |
|---|---|---|---|---|
| 1 | Ever/initial present | 81.3 | | |
| | Present at 4 weeks assess | 51.4 | | |
| | Present at 12 weeks | | | 32.1 |
| 2b | Ever | 27.8 | | |
| | Now | | 15 years | 7.5 |
| 3b | Ever (LE 1 month duration) | 75.8 | | |
| | 1-month duration | 60.6 | | |
| | Within past month | | 12–36 months | 39.4 |
| 3a | 1-month duration | 22.2 | | |
| | Within past month | | 12–36 months | 0.0 |
| 4a | One week | 40.6 | | |
| | Past month | | ≤ 2 years | 24.2 |
| 4b | One week | 62.5 | | |
| | Past month | | ≤ 2 years | 25.8 |
| 5a | One week | 23.4 | | |
| | Past 6 weeks | | 17 years | 5.1 |
| 6 | | 1.0 | | |
| 7 | Recent | | | 70.0 |
| 8 | Current | | 8 months | 48.4 |
| 9 | Current | | | 100 mod/sev |
| 10 | Present 1 month postcrime | | 1 month | 38.4 mod/sev 22.0 mild |
| 11 | 1-month duration | 19.0 | | 5.0 |

*Note.*   Rates based on total sample—not differentiated by crime type.

imately 63% (Study #4b) to over 75% (Studies #1 and #3b) in community agency referred samples. A clear outlier in terms of prevalence is the lowest rate of 1% observed in the Epidemiologic Catchment Area (ECA) study from St. Louis. This discrepancy may relate to sampling as well as other methodological differences.

It appears that rates in community-based samples are lower in general than rates in specially referred samples. In addition, decision rules in all of our samples except Study #2b did not require all symptoms to be specific to trauma. A third difference, however, may relate to assessment of trauma exposure and associated symptoms. The rates of criminal victimization in our samples were higher than those reported in the ECA study. In fact, the highest rates of trauma observed in that study were in association with physical attack, and combat trauma. These exposure types were also apparently the only categories routinely assessed in all subjects. In contrast, with the methodology employed in the other two general community studies, exposure to several types of criminal victimization was routinely assessed. Alternatively, there may be real differences across these samples in terms of victimization rates and/or PTSD rates.

In terms of current PTSD assessed at various periods postcrime, the rates observed in three populations assessed at periods ranging from approximately 10 or more years postcrime ranged form 5% to 7.5%. Rates observed in populations assessed at from 1 to 36 months postcrime generally ranged from 24% or 25% in a criminal justice system (CJS) exposed sample (Studies #4a/4b) to 48.4% (Study #8) and 70% (Study #7) in clinical and crisis agency referred samples, respectively. An exception to this was that no partners of rape victims (Study #3a) met criteria for PTSD at 12- to 36-month assessment.

A further comparison of PTSD rates over time, restricted to samples and subgroups that assessed symptoms among rape victims, can be observed in Table 7–6. Rates under the "initial assessment or symptoms present ever" column indicate a range of rates of PTSD, from 57.1% in a community-based sample to rates of 70% to 95.1% in agency referred samples. At 1 month postrape, the rates ranged from 35% in a community sample to rates around 60% in agency-referred samples.

In Study #1, it can be seen that the rate of PTSD at 12 weeks was less than half as great as the rate at initial assessment. However, this rate of 46%, the rates of 38.4% at 12–36 months in Study #3b, and the rates of 16.5% ob-

Table 7–6.    Longitudinal PTSD rates for rape (percentages)

| Study | Initial (Ever) | Week 4 (1 Month) | Week 6 | Week 8 | Week 12 | 12–36 Months | 15 Years |
|-------|---------|-----------|--------|--------|---------|---------|----------|
| 1     | 95.1    | 63.3      | 59.0   | 52.5   | 45.9    |         |          |
| 2b    | 57.1    |           |        |        |         |         | 16.5     |
| 3b    | 75.8    | 60.6      |        |        |         | 39.4    |          |
| 7     | 70.0    |           |        |        |         |         |          |
| 11    |         | 35.0      |        |        |         |         | 12.5     |

tained in Study #2b and 12.5% in Study #11 after an average of 15 years indicate that PTSD is a chronic disorder for a subset of rape victims. This high rate of PTSD at initial assessment may indicate empirically that rape is the type of stressor that is associated with initial distress in almost everyone. This appears to validate the inclusion of rape as an important potentially traumatic event in Criterion A as it is currently defined. If Criterion A is to be retained, data about the proportion of the general population that does experience at least immediate distress following various types of events would be important empirical information.

## PTSD Rates Associated With Crime Type

Rates of lifetime PTSD associated with a variety of crime types and restricted to direct victims are included in Table 7–7. In this table, rates within samples that had a measure of PTSD at least 1 month postcrime were the lifetime rates used. Within studies that included more than one crime type, there were several significant and fairly consistent findings. In two of the four studies that included these comparisons (Study #1) and (Study #2a), rates of PTSD associated with rape were significantly higher than rates associated with other crimes. In Study #4a, rates associated with rape *and* physical assault were significantly higher than rates associated with other crime. In Study #11, the rates were fairly similar for rape and physical assault—35% and 39%, respectively—and were higher than the rate associated with other sexual assault. In general, the lowest rates of PTSD, ranging from 16.7% to 33%, were associated with the crimes of robbery, burglary, and some nonrape sexual assaults. With the exception of the 3.5% rate observed in Study #6, the lifetime PTSD rates associated with rape, physical attack, and sniper attack ranged from 35% to 70%.

Lifetime PTSD rates associated with indirect victimization are included in Table 7–8. Data related to three major categories—rape or sexual assault of a family member, criminal/vehicular homicide of a family member, and physical assault of a family member, or witnessing a physical assault—were available. Only Study #9 and Study #6 samples contained groups of subjects who had all witnessed the crime. In the sexual assault category, all 10 children who witnessed a mother's assault met PTSD criteria, whereas only 22.2% of a small group of rape victim partners (none of whom was present at assault) and 50% of a criminal justice identified sample had PTSD at some time. The PTSD rates of 23.4% and 24.8% observed in the two community samples in which homicide survivors were assessed (Study #5a and Study #11) were very consistent, while a much higher rate of PTSD (71%) was observed in the sample identified from CJS contact.

Comparisons between criminal and vehicular homicide survivor sub-

Table 7–7.     Lifetime PTSD rates (percentages) by crime type—direct victims

| Study | Rape | Other Sexual Assault | Any Sexual Assault | Physical Assault | Robbery/ Burglary | Crime | Sniper |
|-------|------|------|------|------|------|------|------|
| 1 | 63.3 | | | | | 36.7 | |
| 2a/b | 57.1 | 15.7–33.0 | | 36.8 | 18.2/28.2 | | |
| 3b | 60.6 | | | | | | |
| 4a | | | 68.8 | 58.3 | 27.3/16.7 | | |
| 6 | | | | 3.5 | | | |
| 7 | 70.0 | | | | | | |
| 8 | | | 48.4 | | | | |
| 10 | | | | | | | 38.4 |
| 11 | 35.0 | 23.0 | 29.0 | 39.0 | | | |

**Study 1:** PTSD rate at week 4 significantly higher in rape victim versus general crime victim group, $\chi^2(1) = 7.64$, df = 1 ($N = 112$), $P < .01$. Rape victims also had significantly higher rates of PTSD at initial, 6-week, 8-week, and 12-week assessments.

**Study 2b:** Range of rates for sexual assault: Lowest for attempted rape and highest for completed molestation, with attempted molestation, and other sexual assault intermediate.

Highest lifetime rates for completed rape, aggravated assault, completed molestation, and burglary.

**Study 2a:** Rape only crime type significantly associated with PTSD after controlling for presence of life threat and injury in crime.

**Study 4a:** Overall significant difference by crime type, $\chi^2(3) = 23.11$, df = 3 ($n = 128$), $P < .0005$. PTSD rate in sexual/physical assault subgroup significantly greater than that in robbery/burglary subgroup (60.9% versus 20.3%), $\chi^2(1) = 20.24$, df = 1 ($n = 128$), $P < .0005$.

**Study 11:** Rates of PTSD associated with crimes assessed substantially higher than rates associated with other trauma (detailed in previous table). Lifetime PTSD rate associated with other trauma was 10.0%.

groups indicated no significant differences in PTSD rates associated with type of homicide. Finally, rates associated with witnessing physical assault in a community sample were minimal, whereas a high rate of PTSD (62.5%) was associated with aggravated assault of a family member in the CJS–exposed sample. In general, with the exception of Study #6, the rates of PTSD associated with indirect victimization appear to be comparable with those associated with direct victimization. Analyses comparing rates associated with direct and indirect victims in the CJS–exposed sample indicated no significant differences. Further data on this issue will be available from Study #11 in the future. It is possible that direct and indirect victims in these samples may differ in PTSD symptom patterns, even if differences are not observed at the level of diagnosis. It should be noted, however, that the data on indirect victimization are even more limited than that currently available regarding direct victimization, and these findings must be considered in that light.

## PTSD Associated With Within-Crime Characteristics

Results of chi-square analyses from two samples of PTSD rates associated with presence of the crime characteristics "perceived life threat" and "in-

**Table 7–8.**   Lifetime PTSD rates (percentages) by crime type—indirect victims (witnesses/close family members)

| Study | Rape/Sexual Assault | Criminal/ Vehicular Homicide | Physical Assault |
|-------|---------------------|------------------------------|------------------|
| 3a | 22.2 | | |
| 4b | 50.0 | 71.0 | 62.5 |
| 5a | | 23.4 | |
| 6 | | | 1.7/1.4 per 1,000 M/F |
| 9 | 100.0 | | |
| 11 | | 24.8 | |

*Note.*   Subjects in Study #9 and Study #6 witnessed crime, while subjects in the other studies listed may or may not have been present at scene of crime.
**Study 4b:** Rates not significantly different across crime types, and rates of PTSD associated with indirect victimization not significantly different from rates associated with direct victimization in this sample with high exposure to criminal justice system.
**Study 5a:** Rates associated with criminal or vehicular homicide not significantly different.
**Study 6:** Described as witnessing someone being hurt or killed.
**Study 11:** Rates associated with criminal or vehicular homicide not significantly different.

jury sustained" are included in Table 7–9, along with other findings related to crime characteristics. In both the community and CJS–exposed samples, PTSD rates were significantly associated with the presence of the crime characteristics. In Study #2a, the rates of PTSD were more than doubled if either characteristic was reported, and the rate of 59.2% associated with presence of both life threat and injury was almost 4 times as great as the 14.7% rate observed in the absence of these characteristics. The rates associated with the presence of these features in the community sample were almost identical (65.9%) in both conditions, and the risk ratios associated with their presence were even higher compared to the subgroup in which these features were absent.

An additional finding in this sample was that rape was the only crime type that was significantly associated with PTSD after controlling for presence of life threat and injury, indicating that there may be other aspects to a rape experience that relate to increased risk of PTSD. Findings from other studies indicate that the highest rate of PTSD in the civilian population was associated with physical attack (Study #6) and that physical presence and proximity to the violence were significantly positively associated with num-

---

**Table 7–9.**    Presence of PTSD in association with perceived life threat and injury

| Study | No Life Threat or Injury | Life Threat | Injury | Both | Chi-square |
|---|---|---|---|---|---|
| 2a | 14.7% | 34.5% | 42.9% | 59.2% | $\chi^2(3) = 42.19^*$ |
| 4a | 9.1% | 38.6% | 42.9% | 65.9% | $\chi^2(3) = 25.35^*$ |

* For study #2a, df = 3 ($n = 295$), $P < .0005$; for study #4a, df = 3 ($n = 128$), $P < .0005$.
Consistent findings across two studies, displayed above, indicate higher rates of lifetime PTSD in cases where crime includes life threat or injury. Highest rates observed when both characteristics are present.
**Study 2a:** Results of hierarchical discriminant function analysis indicated significant associations between crime factors of perceived life threat during crime, injury sustained during crime, and crime consisting of completed rape with lifetime PTSD. Only crime of completed rape was significantly associated with PTSD after controlling for presence of the other two crime stress characteristics.
**Study 5:** In homicide survivor group, significantly higher rate of lifetime PTSD observed in subgroup with spouse/sibling/child killed versus subgroup with parent/grandparent/grandchild killed (27.9% versus 12.5%) $\chi^2(1) = 5.02$, df = 1 ($N = 214$), $P < .05$. Lifetime and current search for meaning as to why crime occurred significantly associated with lifetime and current PTSD, respectively.
**Study 6:** Highest rate of PTSD in civilian population associated with physical attack. In veteran population highest rate in subgroup wounded in combat.
**Study 8:** Significantly higher rate of PTSD observed in subgroup sexually abused by natural father (75%) than subgroups in which perpetrator was other trusted adult (25%), or older child (0%).
**Study 10:** Physical presence and proximity to the violence was significantly positively associated with number of PTSD symptoms.

ber of PTSD symptoms following a sniper attack (Study #10).

Other significant findings relate to the relationship with the perpetrator, and for indirect victims, the relationship with the victim. Results from a study of childhood sexual abuse victims (Study #8) indicated that those abused by a natural father had significantly higher rates of PTSD than subjects assaulted by another adult or an older child. Findings in a homicide survivor sample (Study #5) indicated that the rate of PTSD was significantly higher in a subgroup that lost a spouse, sibling, or child to murder than the subgroup in which a parent, grandparent, or grandchild was killed. An additional finding within the homicide survivor group was that persistent lifetime and current search for meaning as to why the crime occurred were significantly positively associated with presence of lifetime and current PTSD, respectively.

One important inference that might be made from some of these findings is that subjective factors such as the perception of serious life threat are very important to our understanding of psychological distress produced by events, perhaps as important as objective indices of threat, including extent of injury sustained. The findings related to quest for meaning and aspects of the rape experience beyond objective and subjective threat in association with PTSD may also be seen as consistent with this concept. This issue also relates to the question of broadening the category of stressors. It is almost certainly the case that there are individual differences in the perceived threat or harm associated with a given event that could then be associated with PTSD symptom patterns and that current definitions of the acceptable stressors are too narrow in this regard.

A further examination of lifetime PTSD symptoms in association with threat and injury is included in Table 7–10. Analyses of variance tests were conducted in two samples (Studies #2 and #4a), to examine the associations between these crime factors and the continuous measures of number of criterion and total PTSD symptoms. The criteria were defined according to DSM-III-R organization for reexperiencing, avoidance, and increased arousal symptoms. Therefore, the two samples differ in the number of total items possible. In Study #2, only the DSM-III (American Psychiatric Association 1980) symptom items were assessed, so a smaller number of criterion and total symptoms were possible. However, the pattern of findings across the two samples appears to be similar. For each criterion and for the total symptom score in both samples, the average number of symptoms was

**Table 7–10.**    Mean number of lifetime criterion items and total PTSD symptoms by threat level

| Criteria | Study | No Life Threat or Injury | Life Threat | Injury | Both | F | P |
|---|---|---|---|---|---|---|---|
| Reexperiencing | 2 | .64 | 1.02 | 1.33 | 1.57 | 13.25 | < .0005 |
|  | 4a | .42 | .91 | 1.00 | 1.80 | 12.39 | < .0005 |
| Avoidance | 2 | .63 | 1.40 | 1.57 | 1.98 | 19.27 | < .0005 |
|  | 4a | 1.36 | 2.36 | 2.86 | 3.52 | 10.20 | < .0005 |
| Arousal | 2 | .65 | 1.04 | 1.71 | 2.31 | 26.08 | < .0005 |
|  | 4a | 2.12 | 3.30 | 3.00 | 4.25 | 6.95 | < .0005 |
| Total PTSD | 2 | 1.92 | 3.45 | 4.62 | 5.86 | 26.72 | < .0005 |
|  | 4a | 3.91 | 6.57 | 6.86 | 9.57 | 11.86 | < .0005 |

*Note.*   Criteria based on DSM-III-R organization. Therefore, number of symptoms per criterion in sample 2 is more limited (3 reexperiencing, 4 arousal, 4 avoidance).

higher in association with threat and injury characteristics present, with the highest number of symptoms present when both characteristics were present. Overall *F*s in every case were highly significant.

## Comorbidity of PTSD With Other Disorders

As inspection of Table 7–11 indicates, the three studies that examined the question of comorbidity all found that individuals with PTSD were at substantially greater risk for also having a variety of other mental disorders. Because all of these samples were non-treatment-seeking in nature, these comorbidity findings are particularly noteworthy. An added feature of Study #2 is a comparison between crime victims with current PTSD, crime victims without current PTSD, and a nonvictimized control group. Statistical comparisons indicated that rates of other disorders in the currently PTSD-negative crime victim group were not significantly different from rates in the noncrime group. Rates of other disorders in the currently PTSD-positive group, however, were significantly higher than rates observed in the other two comparison groups, suggesting that the risk was not due to victimization alone.

In the following comparisons, the risk ratios listed under column (a) (those comparing current PTSD positive to current PTSD negative crime victims) will be referred to. It should be noted that in every case, the risk ratios were even higher in comparison with the noncrime group. In Studies #2 and #6, risk ratios were highest for some of the anxiety disorders and affective disorders. For example, the highest and second-highest increased risk ratios were associated with obsessive-compulsive disorder in Studies #6 and #2, respectively. In these two samples, subjects with PTSD were more than 9 times more likely to also meet criteria for that anxiety disorder as well. The highest risk ratio in Study #2 was associated with agoraphobia, with panic disorder ranked as third in terms of risk ratio.

All three studies assessed comorbidity of PTSD and categories of affective disorder. However, only rates and risk ratios in Studies #2 and #11 are

**Table 7–11.**   Comorbidity of PTSD with other disorders

| | Risk Ratio (With Versus Without PTSD) | | | | | |
|---|---|---|---|---|---|---|
| | Study 2 | | | Study 6 | Study 11 | |
| Other Disorder | a | b | c | | a | b |
| Obsessive-compulsive disorder | 9.4 | 13.0 | 27.3% | 10.1 | 47.1 | |
| Panic disorder | 9.1 | — | 13.6% | 4.0 | | |
| Major depression and/or mania | | | | 5.7 | | |
| Major depressive episode | 7.2 | 31.8 | 31.8% | 14.7 | | |
| Dysthymic disorder | | | | 7.8 | | |
| Phobias | | | | 3.3 | | |
| Social phobia | 3.8 | 8.7 | 18.2% | | | |
| Agoraphobia | 12.1 | 18.2 | 18.2% | | | |
| Antisocial personality | | | | 3.4 | | |
| Drug abuse/dependence | | | | 2.2 | | |
| Alcoholism | | | | 1.6 | | |
| Any core diagnosis | | | | 2.0 | | |
| Sexual dysfunction | 2.1 | 3.6 | 40.9% | | | |

Study 2: Risk ratios under a) above based on current PTSD-positive versus PTSD-negative crime victims. Risk ratios under b) above based on current PTSD-positive versus non-crime victim controls. There were no significant differences between PTSD-negative and non-crime control groups in rates of any disorder. The PTSD-positive group had significantly higher rates of all disorders listed above than both the PTSD-negative and the non-crime control groups. Highest increased risk for agoraphobia, obsessive-compulsive disorder, panic disorder, and major depressive episode. Percentages under c) above are rates of disorder in the current PTSD-positive group.

Study 6: No increased risk for schizophrenia, anorexia nervosa, cognitive impairment. Within male subgroup, no increased risk of phobias or panic. Figures listed in this table are based on total sample (males and females). Greatest increased risk for obsessive-compulsive disorder, dysthymia, and manic-depressive disorder. Unclear whether rates of disorder other than PTSD were based on lifetime or current prevalence. Authors note that presence of any disorder (not PTSD alone) is associated with increased risk of another disorder.

Study 11: a) Risk ratio for currently PTSD-positive versus PTSD-negative. Percentage under b) is rate in current PTSD-positive group. Lifetime rate of depression in currently PTSD-positive group ($N = 51$) was 82.4%; lifetime rate of depression in overall PTSD-negative group ($N = 1,339$) was 23.1%. Overall lifetime prevalence of major depressive episode (MDE) is 30.7%; current rate of MDE is 4.7%.

comparable on the basis of the definitions employed. In these two studies, the presence of current major depressive episode was assessed, whereas in Study #6, one category of affective disorder included major depression and/or mania together. In addition, the presence of dysthymia was also assessed in the latter study. What is comparable across Studies #2 and #5 is the relative ranking of risk ratios for the affective disorder categories. In Study #2, the increased risk for meeting current criteria for major depressive episode followed that associated with the panic and obsessive-compulsive disorders in order of rank. In Study #6, the risk ratios associated with dysthymic disorder and major depression and/or mania followed that associated with obsessive-compulsive disorder in order of rank. Within Study #2 and Study #11 samples, the rates of current depression in subgroups that met criteria for current PTSD were 31.8% and 47.1%, respectively. Those with current PTSD were 7.2 and 14.7 times more likely than subjects without current PTSD to meet current criteria for depression.

In a discussion of the high rates of comorbidity associated with PTSD, Helzer and colleagues (1987) noted that this was also the case for other disorders aside from PTSD. They also raised the issue of the overlap in symptom items included in the diagnostic criteria for the most commonly co-occurring disorders. For example, the symptoms of decreased interest, concentration difficulties, and sleep disturbance are common to both PTSD and major depression. One way to examine this possibility would be to observe patterns of both PTSD and depressive symptoms in groups of patients exposed to potentially traumatic events. Perhaps the overlap in the two disorders might be limited to the shared set of symptoms, or alternatively other patterns might be evident.

Similarly, Helzer and colleagues (1987) noted that obsessive thoughts, or frequent distressing memories of a traumatic event, would be sufficient to meet criteria for obsessive-compulsive disorder. Clinically, we have observed excessive checking behavior as well in some of the crime victim population. It may be that stressors are associated with an increased risk of depressive disorders and other anxiety disorders. It may also be the case that depressive and/or "other" anxiety symptoms associated with trauma may appear to be similar to these syndromes as they are currently classified, but that differences exist in other areas, such as family history or biological correlates. Pitman suggests that indeed there may be important differences in biological correlates such as rapid eye movement (REM) sleep latency that distinguish PTSD from major depressive disorder (see Chapter 9). Finally, the possibility that there may be heterogeneity within the PTSD category, as is recognized with other disorders, should be acknowledged.

Other disorders that were associated with increased risk in the PTSD positive population in Study #6 were drug abuse/dependence and alcoholism. Subjects with PTSD were 2.2 times more likely than others to meet criteria for drug abuse/dependence and 1.6 times more likely to meet criteria for alcoholism. Preliminary data from Study #11 related to comorbidity of individual indices of alcohol abuse and PTSD are presented in Table 7–12. These data are from the national probability sample study of the potential relationships among family history of alcohol/substance abuse, trauma in the family environment, risk of exposure to potentially traumatic events, PTSD, depression, and respondents' use of alcohol and other substances. These data, too, suggest that there is substantial comorbidity between PTSD and substance abuse problems.

Finally, presented in Figure 7–1 are data from a national probability sample of 2,009 women (Study #11a), which depicts comparisons among three groups that differed in terms of exposure to crime and presence or absence

Table 7–12.    Comorbidity of individual indices of alcohol abuse in national sample (percentages, Study #11)

| Indicator | Current PTSD ($n = 46$) | PTSD Lifetime Not Current ($n = 135$) | Non-PTSD ($n = 1,072$) |
|---|---|---|---|
| Trouble at work due to drinking | 11 | 1 | <1 |
| Trouble with friends | 24 | 10 | 4 |
| Driven while under the influence | 48 | 42 | 26 |
| Criticized by family | 22 | 19 | 7 |
| Trouble with police | 11 | 4 | 2 |
| Car accident | 9 | 4 | 1 |
| Home accident | 9 | 4 | 1 |
| Blackout | 33 | 33 | 15 |
| Guzzling for effect | 33 | 18 | 8 |
| Drinking first thing in the morning | 11 | 4 | 1 |
| Couldn't stop drinking | 28 | 16 | 5 |
| Unable to quit or cut down | 15 | 6 | 2 |

*Note.* On alcohol abuse indices, 12.2% of current PTSD subgroup ($n = 51$) were excluded because they reported that they were nondrinkers. In the lifetime but not current PTSD group, 15% of the subgroup ($n = 159$) were excluded for this reason. In the non-PTSD subgroup, 19.9% of the total group ($N = 1,339$) were excluded from further analyses for this reason.

of PTSD, given exposure to crime. All women were separated into three groups based on their crime victim status and whether or not they had ever developed PTSD. Groups included 1) noncrime victims (Non-CV), 2) crime victims without PTSD (CV – PTSD), and 3) crime victims with PTSD (CV + PTSD). The proportion of women in each of these three groups that reported repeated usage and history of *two or more* major alcohol and/or drug-related problems, including problems with work, friends, family, police, and accidents, was determined. As Figure 7–1 indicates, alcohol rather than other drugs was the type of substance with which women reported having the most problems. Results indicated that, irrespective of PTSD status, being a crime victim increased the risk for both serious alcohol and serious drug use problems. In addition, PTSD was a major risk factor for serious substance abuse problems within the crime victim group. Crime victims positive for PTSD were 3.2 times more likely than crime victims without PTSD to have had serious alcohol problems. They were 3.4 times more likely to have serious drug abuse problems. Finally, crime victims with PTSD had a much greater risk than nonvictims of crime of having both types of substance abuse problems. They were 13.7 times more likely than nonvictims to have had major alcohol problems, and they were 22 times more likely than nonvictims to have had major drug abuse problems.

These results indicate that history of criminal victimization increases risk

**Percentage with problems**

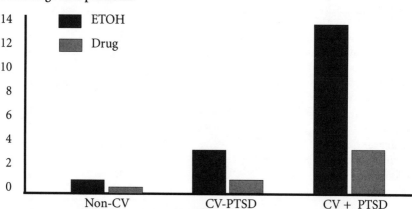

**Figure 7–1.** Women with two or more problems due to substance abuse. ETOH = alcohol; Non-CV = noncrime victims; CV –PTSD = crime victims without PTSD; CV + PTSD = crime victims with PTSD.

for alcohol and drug abuse problems among a national probability sample of adult American women. In addition, it appears that it is the crime victims who experience extreme emotional distress after the crime who are most likely to develop major substance abuse problems. Limitations of the study include the retrospective design. The data indicate increased risk of substance abuse problems associated with PTSD, but causal relationships cannot be inferred.

## Frequencies and Rank Order of Occurrence of Individual Symptoms of PTSD

Table 7–13 includes a listing of lifetime individual PTSD symptoms in three samples (Studies #3b, #4a, and #11). These samples represent a

**Table 7–13.** Lifetime PTSD symptoms from 3 study samples (percentages)

| Lifetime Symptom | 3b ($n = 33$) | 4a ($n = 128$) | 11 (Total $N = 1,101$) |
|---|---|---|---|
| Avoidance of thoughts/feelings | 64 (8) | 65 (2) | 31 (1) |
| Hypervigilance | 88 (2) | 66 (1) | 20 (9) |
| Intrusive memory | 91 (1) | 56 (5) | 24 (6.67) |
| Concentration | 73 (3.67) | 60 (3) | 24 (2) |
| Sleep disturbance | 73 (3.67) | 52 (8) | 29 (2) |
| Irritability | 63 (9) | 40 (11.5) | 27 (3) |
| Startle | 73 (3.67) | 53 (7) | 14 (13) |
| Detachment from others | 70 (6) | 40 (11.5) | 24 (6.67) |
| Decreased interest | 52 (14.5) | 49 (9) | 25 (4.5) |
| Future orientation | 52 (14.5) | 25 (4.5) | |
| Avoidance of activity/situation | 61 (10) | 45 (10) | 17 (11.5) |
| Constricted affect | 36 (16) | 54 (6) | 18 (10) |
| Anxiety reminders | 55 (12.5) | 59 (4) | 10 (17) |
| Mood to reminders | 67 (7) | 12 (16) | |
| Dream/nightmare | 58 (11) | 23 (14) | 13 (14.5) |
| Flashback | 55 (12.5) | 31 (13) | 13 (14.5) |
| Psychogenic amnesia | 27 (17) | 17 (11.5) | |
| **Criteria** | | | |
| Reexperiencing | 97 | 58 | 41 |
| Avoidance | 67 | 52 | 28 |
| Arousal | 91 | 71 | 38 |
| PTSD | 61 | 41 | 19 |

*Note.* In Study #2 sample not included in this table, survivor guilt was assessed. The lifetime prevalence of that symptom was 5.1% in that community sample of crime victims.
Number in parentheses refers to rank order of symptom.

range from a rape crisis center identified population, a sample identified on the basis of CJS contact, and a national probability sample. Rates of symptoms within each group are displayed, as well as the rank order of occurrence of symptoms within each sample. In addition, the average rank order of each symptom was calculated, and the order in which the symptoms are displayed in this table is based on that mean rank in descending order, from avoidance of thoughts or feelings to psychogenic amnesia.

With respect to the mean ranks, it can be noted that the five top-ranked symptoms compose one avoidance, one reexperiencing, and three increased arousal items. Least frequent in terms of mean rank was the symptom of psychogenic amnesia. Although it was not assessed in any of these samples, survivor guilt (Study #2) was the least frequently occurring item in that sample, present in only 5.1% of the crime victim group. The symptom was also rarely observed in Study #6, being present in only 5% of subjects. Constricted affect was also rarely present in that sample. Some of the highest mean rank items listed here were also among the most frequently observed symptoms in the Study #6 sample, including jumpiness and sleep disturbance.

With respect to frequency of occurrence within samples, over 50% of all subjects in the rape crisis center sample displayed each individual symptom, with the exception of constricted affect and psychogenic amnesia. In the CJS sample, at least 40% of all subjects displayed each symptom, with the exception of flashbacks and nightmares. Finally, in the national probability sample, at least 20% of the sample experienced 9 of the individual symptoms, whereas less than that percentage reported avoidance of activities, amnesia, constricted affect, startle, nightmares, flashbacks, dysphoria to reminders, and anxiety to reminders. These eight symptoms also represent items from each of the separate criteria. All symptoms were present in at least 10% of the subsample exposed to potentially traumatic events.

Another observation that can be made from data included in Table 7–13 is that, across samples, the smallest percentage of subjects/respondents met the avoidance criterion for PTSD. An examination of individual symptom rates versus criteria rates suggests that there is some heterogeneity in types of symptoms displayed across the samples. For example, in Study #11, only one of the avoidance items is present in at least 28% of the sample, yet 28% had some combination of three avoidance symptoms. Thus different subjects apparently endorse different symptom items, as opposed to complete homogeneity in the symptom pattern.

## Sensitivity, Specificity, and Predictive Power

The rates of symptoms displayed in Table 7–13 are sensitivity rates. As Widiger and colleagues (1984) have explained, these are actually conditional probabilities that a symptom is present, given the presence of a particular disorder. Similarly, specificity refers to the conditional probability that a symptom is absent in the absence of a particular disorder. As these authors noted, these rates are valuable clinically, in the sense that a symptoms that occurs only rarely would not be useful in prediction. However, another highly informative statistic is the probability of disorder being present or absent, given presence or absence of a particular symptom. Widiger and colleagues labeled these rates positive and negative predictive power, respectively. These rates or probabilities were calculated with the Study #4 data, including the total group of 251 direct and indirect crime victims, and are included in Table 7–14. Rates were calculated for current PTSD. Thus, under the heading +PP, the numbers refer to the probability that a subject meets current criteria for PTSD, given the presence of that particular symptom. Numbers under the –PP heading refer to the probability of not meeting current PTSD criteria, given absence of the particular symptom. The symptoms were ranked in descending order according to the +PP value. In addition, the overall correct classification rate is listed in association with each symptom.

From these data it can be observed that nightmares, the second least frequent symptom with a sensitivity rate of .48, is associated with the highest +PP. Given the presence of dreams or nightmares, there is a .82 probability in this sample of meeting current PTSD criteria. In terms of negative predictive power, the absence of the symptom of recurrent memories is associated with a 1.0 probability that current PTSD is absent. However, given the presence of this symptom, the probability of current PTSD presence is only .56, because this symptom also occurs in the PTSD negative group. In other words, if a person does not have the symptom, he or she does not have PTSD. However, if a person does have the symptom, he or she does not necessarily have PTSD. In terms of overall correct classification, all current symptoms were associated with high classification rates. The highest, 89%, was associated with reduced interest in activities.

Table 7–14.   Conditional probabilities and correct classification rates for current PTSD diagnosis based on presence of individual symptoms in CJS–Exposed Community Sample (Study 4)

| Symptom | Sensitivity | Specificity | +PP | –PP | % Correct |
|---|---|---|---|---|---|
| Nightmares | .48 | .96 | .82 | .85 | .84 |
| Distancing from others | .70 | .93 | .78 | .90 | .87 |
| Reduced interest in activities | .83 | .91 | .77 | .94 | .89 |
| Flashback | .44 | .95 | .74 | .83 | .82 |
| Avoidance of reminders | .73 | .89 | .70 | .91 | .85 |
| Emotional numbing | .85 | .84 | .65 | .95 | .84 |
| Anxiety | .83 | .82 | .62 | .93 | .82 |
| Irritability | .70 | .84 | .60 | .89 | .80 |
| Avoidance/thoughts or feelings | .97 | .75 | .57 | .99 | .80 |
| Concentration | .73 | .81 | .57 | .90 | .79 |
| Startle | .78 | .79 | .56 | .91 | .79 |
| Frequent memories | 1.00 | .73 | .56 | 1.00 | .80 |
| Hypervigilance | .69 | .79 | .53 | .88 | .76 |
| Sleep disturbance | .58 | .81 | .51 | .85 | .75 |

*Note.*   Total sample *N* = 251 (includes direct victims and close family members).

## Numbers of Lifetime PTSD Symptoms in Three Samples

The percentage of subjects in Studies #3b, #4a, and #11 displaying different numbers of each PTSD criterion item are displayed in Table 7–15. The data here are relevant to the issue of cutoff scores used for the criteria. Another important question is the basis upon which this decision rule will be made. The current cutoffs of one reexperiencing symptom, three avoidance symptoms, and two increased arousal symptoms were not empirically derived. One way to examine the relationship of various cutoff scores with diagnosis might be to look at the probability of diagnosis given various patterns or numbers of symptoms, similar to the process described above. It can be observed from Table 7–15 that across samples, the requirement that subjects meet three versus two avoidance items results in a decrease of from 10% to 15% of each sample that meet the criterion. To examine the effects of lowering this criterion to two versus three items, PTSD rates were calculated in two samples using a cutoff of two versus three avoidance symptoms. In Study #3b, the lifetime rate of PTSD with the DSM-III-R cutoff of three was 60.6% for symptoms of 1-month dura-

**Table 7–15.**    Numbers of lifetime DSM-III-R criterion items in three study samples that included DSM-III-R items (percentages)

| Lifetime criterion number | 3b ($n = 33$) | 4a ($n = 128$) | 11 (Total $N = 1{,}101$) |
|---|---|---|---|
| **Reexperiencing** | | | |
| 0 | 3 | 42 | 58 |
| 1 | 12 | 24 | 23 |
| 2 | 30 | 16 | 12 |
| 3 | 18 | 18 | 4 |
| 4 | 36 | | 2 |
| **Avoidance** | | | |
| 0 | 9 | 22 | 37 |
| 1 | 9 | 16 | 21 |
| 2 | 15 | 10 | 14 |
| 3 | 18 | 16 | 11 |
| 4 | 15 | 12 | 7 |
| 5 | 6 | 24 | 5 |
| 6 | 18 | | 4 |
| 7 | 9 | | 1 |
| **Arousal** | | | |
| 0 | 3 | 16 | 45 |
| 1 | 6 | 13 | 18 |
| 2 | 9 | 9 | 15 |
| 3 | 12 | 9 | 10 |
| 4 | 18 | 14 | 7 |
| 5 | 12 | 20 | 4 |
| 6 | 39 | 20 | 2 |

*Note.* One can observe differences in rates of subjects that would meet various criterion item cutoffs. Various cutoff rates could be manipulated to examine differences in full diagnosis rates. In study #3b, in terms of meeting full lifetime diagnostic criteria, analyses indicated that specification of at least 2 versus 3 avoidance items to meet avoidance criterion is associated with a lifetime PTSD rate of 75.8% versus a rate of 60.6%. In study #4a, the rate of lifetime PTSD would be 57.0% versus 40.6%. Analyses for study #11 not yet available.
*Note.* In study #4a, 1 reexperiencing and 2 avoidance items were not included.

tion. With the new cutoff, the rate was 75.8%. The corresponding rates obtained in sample 4a were 40.6% and 57%.

# Recommendations and Conclusions

## Number of Avoidance Symptoms Required to Meet Criteria

We suggest that on the basis of the data, current PTSD symptoms be retained, but that the requirement for meeting the avoidance criterion be reevaluated and possibly lowered from 3 to 2 symptoms to meet criterion.

## Linkage Between Stressor and Symptoms

The present requirement that Criteria B, C, and D symptom items be perceived by the respondent as being specifically related to a specific traumatic event should be evaluated. This requirement seems problematic with respect to avoidance and increased arousal criterion items. In addition, linkage between specific stressor(s) and PTSD symptoms may be especially complicated when there is a history of multiple events. We suggest that guidelines be developed for assessing PTSD in relation to potentially complex event histories.

## Associated Features

Our results suggest that features associated with PTSD include alcohol/substance abuse or dependence. In many instances, symptoms of depression and anxiety may be sufficiently severe to warrant a diagnosis of additional/other anxiety disorders or a depressive disorder.

## Criterion A

Based on the review of the literature in the area of criminal victimization, we propose that Criterion A be broadened to allow for empirical assessment of the potential of a variety of events to elicit distress. Rather than maintaining the current range of acceptable events based on a limited set of predetermined characteristics, this would constitute a more atheoretical descriptive approach. Similarly, we suggest that assumptions should not be made at this time regarding the relationship between the prevalence of a given event (e.g., whether or not it is outside the range of normal human experience) and the likelihood of associated distress. The results of this review indicate that criminal victimization is clearly not outside the range of normal human experience but *is* associated with high rates of PTSD. The data indicate that amongst the population meeting criteria for PTSD, violent crime, particularly for women, is more highly represented than other stressor types than might be expected on the basis of prevalence alone. However, other more commonly experienced events may well be subjectively interpreted as threatening or stressful by those who experience them.

Using the type of empirical approach to identifying criterion events suggested above, the data strongly support the inclusion of rape and other physical assaults as events that *are* markedly distressing to almost anyone. What the data also indicate is that subjective perception of threat is clearly associated with the pattern of reactions currently defined as PTSD. Thus we should not exclude other potentially traumatic events that *appear* to be objectively less threatening on an a priori basis.

Resolution of many of the conceptual, methodological, and political problems surrounding the diagnosis of PTSD could be accomplished by the following strategy:

1. Systematically collect detailed information from all individuals about potentially traumatic life events they might have experienced, including events currently listed in Criterion A, as well as other events that are sometimes perceived as distressing.
2. Ask individuals who have experienced each event to rate the level of distress it produced.
3. Collect information on PTSD symptoms, as well as symptoms of other mental health disorders which each person experienced postevent.
4. Determine the probability that given stressful events were associated with PTSD, PTSD symptoms, and/or with other disorders.

This strategy would yield normative data on the prevalence of potentially stressful events, on how distressing they generally are to most people, and on the types of PTSD and other symptoms that are most likely to result from their occurrence. Implicit in the definition of events that are included in Criterion A are the relative prevalence of events (e.g., are they outside the range of normal human experience) and of the relative extent to which we think they should be experienced as distressing (e.g., events that would be markedly distressing to almost anyone). Without empirical information on the prevalence of events and how distressing most people find them, it is totally impossible to empirically determine whether reactions to those events are disorders or merely normal reactions to extraordinary stressful situations.

# References

American Psychiatric Association: Diagnostic and Statistical Manual of Mental Disorders, 3rd Edition. Washington, DC, American Psychiatric Association, 1980

American Psychiatric Association: Diagnostic and Statistical Manual of Mental Disorders, 3rd Edition, Revised. Washington, DC, American Psychiatric Association, 1987

Amick AE, Kilpatrick DG, Resnick HS, et al: Public health implications of homicide for surviving family members: An epidemiological study. Paper presented at the Society of Behavioral Medicine Meeting, San Francisco, CA, April 1989

Foa EB, Rothbaum BO: Rape and crime victims response study. NIMH Grant Number: MH29602. Unpublished manuscript, 1989

Frank E, Anderson BP: Psychiatric disorders in rape victims: Past history and current symptomatology. Compr Psychiatry 28:77–82, 1987

Green BL: Defining trauma: Terminology and generic stressor dimensions. Journal of Applied Social Psychology 20:1632–1642, 1990

Helzer JE, Robins LN, McEvoy L: Post-traumatic stress disorder in the general population. N Engl J Med 317:1630–1634, 1987

Kilpatrick DG: Violence as a precursor of women's substance abuse: The rest of the drug-violence story. Paper presented at Topical Mini-Convention on Substance Abuse and Violence at the 98th Annual Convention of the American Psychological Association, Boston, MA, August 1990

Kilpatrick DG, Saunders BE, Veronen LJ, et al; Criminal victimization: Lifetime prevalence, reporting to police, and psychological impact. Crime and Delinquency 33:479–489, 1987a

Kilpatrick DG, Veronen LJ, Saunders BE, et al: The psychological impact of crime: a study of randomly surveyed crime victims. Final Report, National Institute of Justice Grant No.: 84-IJ-CX-0039, 1987b

Kilpatrick DG, Tidwell RP, Walker E, et al: Victim rights and services in South Carolina: the dream, the law, the reality. Final Report, Justice Assistance Act Grant No.: 86-024, 1989a

Kilpatrick DG, Saunders BE, Amick-McMullan A, et al: Victim and crime factors associated with the development of crime-related post-traumatic stress disorder. Behavior Therapy 20:199–214, 1989b

Kilpatrick DG, Resnick HS, Amick A: Family members of homicide victims: Search for meaning and post-traumatic stress disorder. Paper presented at the 97th Annual Convention of the American Psychological Association, New Orleans, LA, August 1989c

Kilpatrick DG, Best C, Amick-McMullan A, et al: Criminal victimization, post-traumatic stress disorder, and substance abuse: a prospective study, in Comorbidity in Traumatic Stress Disorder With Special Attention to Substance Abuse and Dependence. Chaired by Abueg FR. Symposium conducted at the 23rd Annual Convention of the Association for Advancement of Behavior Therapy, Washington, DC, November 1989d

Kilpatrick DG, Amick AA, Resnick HS: The impact of homicide on surviving family members. Final Report, National Institute of Justice Grant No: 87-IJ-CX-0017, 1990

McLeer SV, Deblinger E, Atkins MS, et al: Post-traumatic stress disorder in sexually abused children. J Am Acad Child Adolesc Psychiatry 27:650–654, 1988

Pynoos RS, Nader K: Children who witness the sexual assaults of their mothers. J Am Acad Child Adolesc Psychiatry 27:567–572, 1988

Pynoos RS, Frederick C, Nader K, et al: Life threat and posttraumatic stress in school-age children. Arch Gen Psychiatry 44:1057–1063, 1987

Resnick HS, Veronen LJ, Saunders BE: Symptoms of PTSD in rape victims and their partners: a behavioral formulation, in The Impact of Rape on Family Functioning: Empirical Findings and Treatment Implications. Chaired by Resick P. Panel conducted at the meeting of the Society for Traumatic Stress Studies, Dallas, TX, October 1988

Resnick HS, Veronen LJ, Saunders BE, et al: Assessment of PTSD in a subset of rape victims at 12 to 36 months post-assault. Unpublished manuscript, 1989

Rothbaum BO, Foa EB, Hoge LA: Responses following sexual and non-sexual assault. Paper presented at the 22nd Annual Convention of the Association for the Advancement of Behavior Therapy, New York, November 1988

Solomon SD, Canino GJ: Appropriateness of DSM-III-R criteria for post-traumatic stress disorder. Compr Psychiatry 31:227–237, 1990

Veronen LJ, Saunders BE: The impact of rape on dyadic involvement and functioning. NIMH Grant No.: 1R01-MH40360, 1989

Widiger TA, Hurst SW, Frances A, et al: Diagnostic efficiency and DSM-III. Arch Gen Psychiatry 41:1005–1012, 1984

◆

# Section III:

# Posttraumatic Stress Disorder in the Community: Prevalence, Features, and Risk Factors

◆

# ◆ 8 ◆ The Epidemiology of Posttraumatic Stress Disorder

Jonathan R. T. Davidson, M.D.
John A. Fairbank, Ph.D.

***Summary***     There has been growing interest in the epidemiology of posttraumatic stress disorder (PTSD). The authors review several studies, grouped into high-risk cohorts (e.g., combat veterans, victims of disaster) and non-high-risk general population samples. They evaluate prevalence rates, rates of chronicity, comorbidity patterns, pretrauma and trauma risk factors, interactive trauma risk factors, and characteristic symptomatology. Finally, they assemble evidence to support the uniqueness of the underlying construct that PTSD differs from other major disorders in its relationship to a traumatic event.

## Statement of the Issue

Epidemiology is the study of the distribution and determinants of health-related states and events in populations (Last 1983). Population-based studies of PTSD are important for formulating unbiased estimates of prevalence and risk factors (Kulka and Schlenger, in press; Weissman et al. 1986). Characterizing PTSD solely on the basis of treatment-seeking samples excludes from study a large proportion of the population with this disorder. McFarlane's (1988a) community-based study of Australian fire fighters provides a striking example of the importance of population-based studies of PTSD. Of the 20 PTSD cases in McFarlane's sample, only one had previously sought mental health treatment, leading the author to suggest that samples drawn from treatment populations may in fact be somewhat atypical of the total population of people with PTSD.

147

We reviewed two kinds of population-based studies of PTSD: populations at risk (e.g., combat veterans, disaster victims) and general population samples. Some of the studies in this review sampled both groups. In this chapter, we report on studies that have examined the following issues:

1. Lifetime and current prevalence of PTSD;
2. Duration of PTSD symptoms;
3. Comorbidity patterns;
4. Pretrauma risk factors for PTSD;
5. Characteristics of extreme events (e.g., intensity) as predictors of PTSD;
6. Pretrauma risk factor (premorbid vulnerability) by trauma interactions;
7. Characteristic symptomatology of PTSD;
8. Differences between acute and chronic PTSD; and
9. Specificity of the trauma-PTSD connection as a validator of PTSD.

# Lifetime and Current Prevalence

We discuss lifetime and current prevalence by focusing on three types of studies: 1) community-based surveys, 2) surveys of nonmilitary at-risk groups, and 3) studies of Vietnam War veterans.

## Community-Based Studies

Table 8–1 describes the lifetime prevalence values for PTSD. Three studies have used the Diagnostic Interview Schedule (DIS; Robins et al. 1981) for diagnosing PTSD in the general population. The DIS is a highly structured survey interview instrument designed specifically for use by lay interviewers (i.e., interviewers without formal clinical training). In the St. Louis site of the Epidemiologic Catchment Area (ECA) survey, Helzer and colleagues (1987) interviewed respondents using the DIS and found a 1% lifetime prevalence of PTSD in the general adult population of the St. Louis metropolitan area. Using the DIS in the North Carolina ECA survey site, we reported a 1.3% lifetime prevalence among adults in the Piedmont region of North Carolina (Davidson et al. 1991). The St. Louis and North Carolina studies also surveyed individuals exposed to a specific trauma using DSM-III diagnostic criteria (American Psychiatric Association 1980). In a small sample of 64 combat veterans in St. Louis, the lifetime prevalence of PTSD was 6.3% (Helzer et al. 1987), and the lifetime prevalence following sexual assault in the North Carolina study was 3.3% (Winfield et al. 1990). Although the St. Louis and North Carolina ECA

**Table 8–1.**   Prevalence rates (percentages) of PTSD in different populations

| Investigator | Population | Lifetime | Current | Instrument |
|---|---|---|---|---|
| Helzer et al. 1987 | ECA—St. Louis | 1.0 | | DIS |
| Davidson et al. 1991 | ECA—Piedmont NC | 1.3 | | DIS |
| Shore et al. 1989 | Mount St. Helens | | | |
| | At Risk | 3.6 | — | DIS |
| | Control | 2.6 | — | |
| | Total | 3.1 | — | |
| Card 1987 | Vietnam Veterans | — | 19.3 | Questionnaire |
| | Veterans of other wars | — | 12.9 | |
| | Nonveterans | — | 12.1 | |
| McFarlane 1989 | Fire Fighters | — | 27-32 | GHQ |
| Pynoos et al. 1987 | Schoolchildren | — | 58.4 | PTSD Index |
| CDC's VES 1988 | Vietnam Veterans | | | |
| | Combat | 14.7 | 2.2 | DIS |
| | Other | 1.8 | — | |
| | Veterans of other wars | | | |
| | Combat | 0.6 | — | |
| | Other | 2.6 | — | |
| Breslau et al. 1991 | HMO Cohort of Young Adults | | | |
| | Total | 9.2 | — | DIS |
| | At Risk | 24.0 | — | (DSM-III-R) |
| Kilpatrick et al.[a] | Community Sample | 27.8 | 7.5 | DIS |
| Veronen et al.[b] | Rape Victims | 75.8 | 39.4 | SCID (DSM-III-R) |
| Kilpatrick et al.[c] | National | | | DIS |
| | Random Sample | 19.0 | 5.0 | (DSM-III-R) |
| Goldberg et al. 1990 | Vietnam Twin | | 5.1[d] | DSM-III-R |
| | Registry | | 5.0[e] | Health |
| | (MZ Twins) | | 16.8[f] | Survey |
| | | | 12.9[g] | |

*Note.*   CDC's VES = Center for Disease Control Vietnam Experience Study; DIS = Diagnostic Interview Schedule (DSM-III criteria unless otherwise specified); DSM-III-R = *Diagnostic and Statistical Manual, 3rd Edition, Revised*; ECA = Epidemiologic Catchment Area Study; GHQ = General Health Questionnaire; HMO = health maintenance organization; MZ = monozygotic; SCID = Structured Clinical Interview for DSM-III.
[a] Kilpatrick D, The psychological impact of crime (unpublished, 1987).
[b] Veronen LJ, Rape relationship project (unpublished, 1989).
[c] Kilpatrick DG, Risk factors for substance abuse: a longitudinal study (unpublished,1989).
[d] Neither twin served in Southeast Asia.
[e] Pair discordant for service: did not serve in Southeast Asia.
[f] Pair discordant for service: served in Southeast Asia.
[g] Both twins served in Southeast Asia.

estimates of PTSD in high-risk groups are of interest, the reliability and generalizability of these estimates are doubtful because the samples were small and geographically limited.

Breslau and colleagues (1991) studied prevalence of exposure to trauma, and of the PTSD diagnosis, in a health maintenance organization (HMO)–enrolled cohort of young adults in Detroit. They found a 9% lifetime prevalence of PTSD, a figure that rose to 24% among those individuals who had been trauma victims. This study employed the DIS to evaluate for PTSD, according to DSM-III-R criteria (American Psychiatric Association 1987).

## Surveys of Nonmilitary At-Risk Groups

A report by Shore and colleagues (1989) addressed PTSD in the population exposed to the Mount St. Helens (MSH) volcanic eruption, as well as a control group who were unexposed to the effects of this natural disaster. Base lifetime prevalence rates were 3.6% in the MSH group and 2.6% in the control group, with a 3.1% overall lifetime prevalence. There thus appears to be an impressive consistency in DIS-based lifetime prevalence rates of PTSD, ranging from 1.0% to 2.6% in the general population and rising to 3.3% to 6.3% in various risk groups exposed to unusual and distressing trauma.

A study by McFarlane (1989) assessed PTSD among a sample of 315 fire fighters of an Australian brushfire using the General Health Questionnaire (GHQ; Goldberg 1972). The GHQ had been validated as a screening instrument for PTSD using a structured clinical interview designed to diagnose PTSD (McFarlane 1989). Prevalence rates of 32%, 27%, and 30% were obtained at 4, 11, and 29 months postexposure, respectively. The appropriateness of the GHQ-based diagnosis of PTSD used in this study is unclear. A subgroup of 49 subjects from McFarlane's study, however, were assessed for PTSD using a structured clinical interview; 34 of these were assessed with the DIS. The prevalence rate of PTSD in these samples was found to be 18% at 8 months using the structured interview (increasing to 28% if partial cases were included) and 35% at 42 months using the DIS. Such rates provide some evidence of the GHQ's usefulness as a screening instrument for PTSD.

Kilpatrick and Resnick (Chapter 7) found lifetime prevalence rates of PTSD among crime victims to vary from 19% to 75% and current prevalence rates to vary from 5% to 39%. DSM-III-R criteria were used in two of their three studies.

In a study of schoolchildren exposed to a sniper attack, Pynoos and associates (1987) observed a 58.4% prevalence of acute PTSD 1 month after the attack. Their sample of 159 children was obtained at random from a total school population of 1,100. PTSD was diagnosed in this study by the PTSD Index interview.

## Surveys of Vietnam Veterans At-Risk Groups

Card (1987) conducted a 21-year follow-up study of a national cohort of 1.1 million ninth graders originally sampled in 1960. Out of a sample of 1,500, 481 were Vietnam veterans, 502 were veterans of other wars, and 487 were nonveterans. Because the data collection component of this study was implemented prior to the publication of the official diagnostic criteria for PTSD in 1989, Card employed a diagnostic algorithm, based on a partial reconstruction of items that approximates DSM-III criteria, to estimate PTSD prevalence. The lifetime prevalence of PTSD in the three groups was 19.3% (Vietnam veterans), 12.9% (veterans of other wars), and 12.1% (nonveterans). However, it is difficult to determine the relationship of these estimates to the prevalence of PTSD as defined by DSM-III or DSM-III-R.

Based on a mail survey of Vietnam veterans selected from lists of American Legion members in six specific states, Snow and associates (1988) reported current PTSD prevalence rates ranging from 1.8% to 15%, depending on how the concept of exposure to war zone stress was operationalized. However, the generalizability of the Legion study findings is limited by several factors. First, the estimates were reported for Vietnam veterans who belonged to the American Legion. There may also be important demographic and other differences between Vietnam veterans who belong to veterans' organizations and those who do not. Second, the relatively low response rates raise concern over the potential impact of nonresponse bias on the estimates. Third, prevalence estimates were based on a single self-report instrument, and the relationship between diagnoses based on that instrument and those based on other methods of diagnosis is unknown.

The Centers for Disease Control (CDC; 1988) published findings from the Vietnam Experience Study (VES), which is one component of a comprehensive, congressionally mandated study of the health effects of military service in Vietnam. In the VES, a random subsample of 2,490 Vietnam veterans was selected from a larger sample of enlisted men who had entered the U.S. Army between 1965 and 1972. Using a slightly modified version of the DIS, the CDC research team estimated that approximately 15% of these veterans had experienced combat-related PTSD at some time during or after their military service and that the prevalence of the disorder during the 1 month prior to the assessment was 2.2%.

Also, Kulka and colleagues (1990) reported PTSD prevalence findings from a nationally representative study of Vietnam veterans, the National Vietnam Veterans Readjustment Study (NVVRS). These estimates are shown in Table 8–2. The NVVRS research design included face-to-face interviews with representative samples of men and women who served in the U.S. Armed Forces in Vietnam, Cambodia, or Laos (Vietnam-theater veterans); men and women who served in the U.S. military during the Vietnam era but not in Southeast Asia (Vietnam-era veterans); and civilian counterparts. A total of 3,016 interviews were conducted throughout the 50 states and Puerto Rico. PTSD prevalence estimates were made using a multimeasure PTSD assessment procedure that included a structured clinical inter-

**Table 8–2.**    NVVRS estimates of current PTSD prevalence[a]—percentages by study group (standard errors in parentheses)

| Study Group | Current PTSD Men | Prevalence Women |
|---|---|---|
| Theater veterans | 15.2 (1.1) | 8.5 (1.1) |
| War zone stress exposure subgroups: | | |
| High | 38.5 (2.8) | 17.5 (2.3) |
| Low/moderate | 8.5 (0.9) | 2.5 (0.6) |
| Race/ethnicity subgroups: | | |
| White/other | 13.7 (1.2) | — |
| Black | 20.6 (2.0) | — |
| Hispanic | 27.9 (2.5) | — |
| Era veterans | | |
| Standardized to theater veterans | 2.5 (0.7) | 1.1 (0.6) |
| Standardized to HWZ theater veterans | 2.8 (0.7) | 1.1 (0.7) |
| Civilian counterparts | | |
| Standardized to theater veterans | 1.2 (0.4) | 0.3 (0.1) |
| Standardized to HWZ theater veterans | 1.3 (0.4) | 0.3 (0.1) |

*Note.*  HWZ = high war zone stressor exposure; NVVRS = National Vietnam Veterans Readjustment Study; PTSD = posttraumatic stress disorder.
[a]*Source:*  Kulka et al. 1990.

view (Spitzer et al. 1987), a clinician rating scale (Weiss et al. 1984), and self-report inventories (Horowitz et al. 1979; Keane et al. 1984, 1988). The NVVRS findings indicated that 15.2% of male and 8.5% of female Vietnam-theater veterans met DSM-III-R diagnostic criteria for PTSD within 6 months of the assessment. These estimates suggested that approximately 480,000 of the 3.2 million veterans who served in the Vietnam theater had PTSD in 1988. For both sexes, current PTSD prevalence rates for Vietnam-theater veterans were consistently higher than rates for Vietnam-era veterans (current prevalence of 2.5% male, 1.1% female) or civilian counterparts (1.2% male, 0.3% female).

The NVVRS findings also indicated that the lifetime prevalence of PTSD was 30.9% among males and 26.9% among female Vietnam-theater veterans. The NVVRS also reported estimates for current "partial PTSD" among Vietnam-theater veterans. Specifically, 11.1% of male and 7.8% of female Vietnam-theater veterans had significant partial symptomatology during the 6 months that preceded the NVVRS interviews.

The disparity between the NVVRS and VES findings on the current prevalence of PTSD (15.2% versus 2.2%) among Vietnam veterans is striking. Although the evidence is not complete, analyses of NVVRS data have suggested that the major contributing factor to this difference was the methods used for PTSD case determination in the two studies (Kulka et al. 1990). PTSD cases were identified in the VES using the DIS administered by trained lay interviewers. Cases in the NVVRS were identified by their agreement over multiple measures of PTSD, including a self-administered Minnesota Multiphasic Personality Inventory (MMPI; Hathaway and McKinley 1989), reports of symptoms to lay interviewers using the Mississippi Scale for Combat-Related PTSD (Keane et al. 1988), and the judgment of highly trained expert clinicians. Analyses of NVVRS data have also suggested that the DIS-like PTSD assessment instrument identified only one in four of even the most severe current cases of PTSD, indicating a degree of sensitivity insufficient to detect true PTSD cases in a community population.

Goldberg and colleagues (1990) reported on a series of male monozygotic twins who had served in the military between 1965 and 1975. In 4,184 twins, the current PTSD prevalence rates were 5.1%, 5.0%, 16.8%, and 12.9%, respectively, for the following groups: 1) those where neither twin served in SEA (Southeast Asia); 2) those of the twin who did not serve in SEA in a pair discordant for SEA duty; 3) those of the twin who served in

SEA in the same discordant pair; and 4) those where both twins served in SEA. Prevalence rates for PTSD also rose with the level of combat exposure. These results indicated that, when possible variance due to genetic and early environmental factors was kept constant, the risk of developing PTSD was proportional to the intensity of exposure to trauma. No other epidemiological or risk factor study of PTSD has controlled for genetic factors, making the report by Goldberg and colleagues unique. Nevertheless, the study does have some limitations, as acknowledged by the authors.

In addition to these reviews, we also wish to note that the lifetime prevalence rates of partial (i.e., subthreshold) forms of PTSD were 6.6% in the North Carolina ECA, 15% in the St. Louis ECA, and 21.2% (females) and 22.5% (males) in the NVVRS (Table 8–3). These findings suggest that a spectrum of PTSD reactions is common in the general population and may occur among 50% or more of such at-risk populations as combat veterans.

# Duration of PTSD Symptoms in Relationship to Trauma

Comparison of current and lifetime PTSD prevalence rates in the NVVRS (Kulka et al. 1990) indicated that 49.2% of the male Vietnam-theater veterans and 31.6% of the female veterans who had ever had PTSD still had it in 1988. In the St. Louis ECA study (Helzer et al. 1987), 49% of PTSD subjects had symptoms that were resolved within 6 months and 51% of the group had symptoms that persisted beyond 6 months, with 33% of the full PTSD population having symptoms lasting beyond 36 months. Chronicity was also found in the North Carolina ECA study (Davidson et al. 1991): Symptoms lasted for less than 1 month in 30%, 1 to 6 months in 16%, 6 to 12 months in 7%, and more than 12 months in 47% of the subjects.

**Table 8–3.**     Lifetime prevalence of symptoms of partial PTSD (percentages)

| Population | Investigators | Prevalence | Instrument |
|---|---|---|---|
| ECA | Helzer et al. 1987 | 15.0 | DIS |
| ECA | Davidson et al. 1991 | 6.6 | DIS |
| NVVRS | Kulka et al. 1990 | | |
| | Males | 22.5 | Composite: |
| | Females | 21.2 | Multiple scales |

*Note.* ECA = Epidemiologic Catchment Area Study; DIS = Diagnostic Interview Schedule; NVVRS = National Vietnam Veterans Readjustment Study.

There is also some evidence that persistence of symptoms is related to the type of trauma. In the St. Louis ECA study (Helzer et al. 1987), combat and physical attack were commonly associated with symptoms lasting beyond 3 years, with chronicity occurring in 53% of combat veterans and 41% of women who had been physically attacked. In the North Carolina ECA study (Davidson et al. 1991), chronic PTSD was more frequently found in patients who had been attacked physically, had been in combat, or had seen someone hurt or killed. Events described as "something else" were found more often to be self-limiting acute cases.

In the Card study (1987), all cases were chronic in that symptoms were assessed as present at the time of examination. McFarlane (1988b) found that 49.8% of his sample met criteria for PTSD at some time during a 29-month follow-up study: 21% manifested a chronic form of PTSD, 9.2% manifested an acute PTSD, and 19.7% manifested a delayed PTSD. Of the chronic group, only 27.2% (18 out of 66) ultimately experienced a resolution of symptoms.

In their studies, Shore and colleagues (Shore 1986; Shore et al. 1986b, 1989) noted that PTSD was the most severe and persistent of the three MSH stress disorders (depression, generalized anxiety disorder [GAD], and PTSD). Although spontaneous remission appeared not to be the general rule, findings from the CDC's VES (1988) stood in marked contrast to this trend, because they indicated a lifetime PTSD prevalence of 15% and a current prevalence of 2.2%, thus suggesting that PTSD was a relatively time-limited disorder. Possible reasons for this anomalous finding related to assessment methods have been suggested (Kulka et al., in press).

Overall, however, most epidemiological findings are consistent with the conceptualization of PTSD as a chronic disorder, rather than an acute or self-limited one. Given that PTSD appears to have a high propensity for chronicity, it would not be surprising if predictors of chronic PTSD might go beyond the simple impact of the trauma itself (this is reviewed below) and be influenced by other factors associated with chronic mental disorder.

## Comorbidity Patterns

The literature on patient populations indicated a high degree of comorbidity (Table 8–4). Our review of the general population-based samples indicated that comorbidity also occurred in a high proportion of people with PTSD. In the St. Louis ECA study (Helzer et al. 1987), almost 80% of full PTSD cases had a previous or concurrent psychiatric disorder, compared to about one-third in respondents with no posttraumatic distress symptoms. In the North Carolina ECA study (Davidson et al. 1991), 62% of individuals with PTSD had a lifetime comorbidity of a psychiatric illness as compared to only 15% of the control group. Ninety-two percent of the MSH PTSD group had comorbidity with PTSD.

The NVVRS (Kulka et al. 1990) found similarly high rates of psychiatric comorbidity among Vietnam veterans with PTSD (Table 8–5). In this study, 50% of Vietnam-theater veterans with current PTSD also met criteria for at least one other DSM-III-based psychological disorder within the 6 months prior to assessment, compared to 11.5% of Vietnam-theater veterans without a current diagnosis of PTSD. As expected, lifetime PTSD comorbidities among Vietnam-theater veterans were even higher. Virtually all (98.8%) theater veterans with current PTSD (as of 1988) were found to have met the criteria for at least one other psychiatric disorder (including substance abuse and dependence) at some time during their lives. The NVVRS findings on the co-occurrence of specific current and lifetime psychiatric disorders with PTSD are shown in Table 8–5. With regard to some specific affective disorders, for example, the NVVRS reported that 15.7% of male

**Table 8–4.**    Comorbidity with PTSD

| North Carolina ECA[a] | | Panic disorder | (4.0) |
|---|---|---|---|
| Somatization disorder | (90.2) | Antisocial personality disorder | (3.4) |
| Schizophrenia | (37.0) | Phobias (combined) | (3.3) |
| Panic disorder | (21.2) | Drug abuse | (2.2) |
| Social phobia | (13.9) | Alcohol abuse | (1.6) |
| Obsessive-compulsive disorder | (11.9) | **Mount St. Helens Study[c]** | |
| Generalized anxiety disorder | (11.1) | Generalized anxiety disorder | (76%) |
| Depression | (11.0) | Depression | (51%) |
| Drug abuse | (9.8) | Phobias | (35%) |
| Simple phobia | (9.0) | Alcohol abuse | (27%) |
| Agoraphobia | (8.4) | Obsessive-compulsive disorder | (11%) |
| **St. Louis ECA[b]** | | Drug abuse | (8%) |
| Obsessive-compulsive disorder | (10.1) | Panic disorder | (8%) |
| Dysthymia | (7.8) | Mania | (5%) |
| Manic depression | (5.7) | Antisocial personality disorder | (5%) |

[a] Lifetime figures refer to odds ratio relative to control.
[b] Lifetime figures refer to increased risk relative to control.
[c] Concurrent percentage frequency within PTSD group.

Vietnam-theater veterans and 23% of female theater veterans with current PTSD had experienced a recent major depressive episode; 4.4% of the men and 2.5% of the women had experienced a manic episode during the 6 months preceding the interview. In the NVVRS (Kulka et al. 1990), alcohol abuse, major depression, and GAD were the most common comorbid disorders among men; depression, GAD, alcohol abuse, and panic disorder were the most common comorbid disorders among women.

The CDC's (1988) VES also reported high rates of co-occurring depression, GAD, and substance abuse among Vietnam veterans with PTSD relative to veterans without this disorder. For example, as shown in Table 8–5, 17.5% of Vietnam-theater veterans who had ever met the criteria for PTSD also met the criteria for depression during the month preceding the VES evaluation. This estimate of the prevalence of co-occurring depression is significantly greater than the rate of 2.3% found among Vietnam-theater veterans who had never met the criteria for a PTSD diagnosis. Thus, in the Vietnam veteran population, solitary PTSD was uncommon.

Of particular interest to the diagnostic nature of PTSD was the finding in the North Carolina ECA study (Davidson et al. 1991) that highest risk was found for associations between PTSD and somatization disorder and

**Table 8–5.** Lifetime and current comorbidity in NVVRS and CDC's VES studies (percentages)

| | NVVRS Theater Veterans | | | | CDC's VES | |
| | Men | | Women | | | |
| | Previous 6 Months | Ever | Previous 6 Months | Ever | Previous Month | Ever |
|---|---|---|---|---|---|---|
| Major depression | 15.7 | 26.4 | 23.0 | 42.3 | 17.5 | 34.2 |
| Mania | 4.4 | 5.5 | 2.5 | 2.5 | — | — |
| Dysthymia | — | 21.0 | — | 33.2 | — | — |
| Panic disorder | 4.9 | 8.0 | 12.7 | 20.8 | — | — |
| Obsessive-compulsive disorder | 8.7 | 10.4 | 7.5 | 12.7 | — | — |
| Generalized anxiety disorder | 19.8 | 43.5 | 19.4 | 38.2 | 14.2 | 45.1 |
| Alcohol abuse | 22.2 | 73.8 | 10.1 | 28.5 | | 70.0 |
| Drug abuse | 6.1 | 11.3 | <1.0 | 8.0 | 26.2 | 25.4 |
| Antisocial personality | 10.8 | — | <1.0 | — | — | — |

*Note.* CDC's VES = Centers for Disease Control Vietnam Experience Study; NVVRS = National Vietnam Veterans Readjustment Study.
*Source.* Kulka et al. 1990.

between PTSD and schizophrenia/schizophreniform disorder. The high comorbidity with somatization disorder suggested that dissociative and conversion mechanisms were indeed characteristic elements of PTSD. They also accorded, by an entirely different methodological approach, with Briquet's clinical observations made more than 100 years ago in Europe that somatization disorder frequently occurred in victims of early trauma (Mai and Merskey 1980).

As noted by several investigators (Keane and Wolfe 1990; Kulka et al. 1990), the issue of cause and effect regarding the broad spectrum of co-occurring disorders in individuals with PTSD is as yet unresolved. Research is needed to determine if exposure to extreme stress produces the range of co-occurring disorders observed among individuals with PTSD, or if the presence of other psychiatric disorders increases a person's risk for developing PTSD following exposure to extreme events.

# Pretrauma Risk Factors for PTSD

Some studies (Table 8–6) have found evidence of pretrauma risk factors. Such factors include familial psychiatric illness; parental poverty; childhood trauma (e.g., sexual assault, separated or divorced parents before age 10; Davidson et al. 1991); childhood behavior disorder (Helzer et al. 1987); poor self-confidence at age 15 (Card 1987); neuroticism; introversion; prior psychiatric disorder; adverse life events before and after the trauma (McFarlane 1989); being female and between ages 36 and 50; being concerned about finances and having prior physical health problems (Shore et al. 1986a); meeting the criteria for conduct disorder; growing up in a family with economic problems; and having a relative with major mental disorder (Kulka et al. 1990). In the MSH survey, women but not men with preexisting GAD and depression were at risk to a recurrence following exposure to trauma.

Helzer and colleagues (1987) noted that a premorbid risk factor increased the risk of exposure to trauma and the risk of developing symptoms from the event. Davidson and colleagues (1991) controlled for other psychiatric disorders and found that only parental poverty continued to exert a statistically significant effect, increasing the chance of PTSD.

**Table 8–6.** Premorbid risk factors for PTSD

| Study | Risk Factors | Comments |
|-------|-------------|----------|
| Davidson et al. 1991 | Familial psychiatric illness<br>Parental poverty<br>Abused as child<br>Sexual assault before age 16<br>Separation/divorce of patients < age 10<br>Female | After controlling for comorbidity, only parental poverty remained significant |
| Helzer et al. 1987 | Childhood behavior disorder<br>Female | Increased risk for exposure to trauma and for developing symptoms |
| Card 1987 | Poor self confidence at age 15 | |
| Shore et al. 1986a, 1986b, 1989 | Females aged 36–50<br>Concern over finances<br>Prior physical illness | Premorbid risk factor more evident at lower levels of exposure intensity |
| McFarlane 1989 | Neuroticism<br>Introversion<br>Previous psychiatric disorder<br>Adverse life events prior to trauma<br>Postdisaster life events | 4, 11, 29 months<br>4 months<br>4, 29 months<br>4 months<br>11 and 29 months |
| Kulka et al. 1990 | Number of behavior problems in childhood<br>Meeting criteria for conduct disorder<br>Growing up in a family with economic problems<br>Having one or more first degree relatives with a mental disorder | |
| Breslau et al. 1991 | Neuroticism<br>Early separation from parents<br>Family history of anxiety<br>Low education<br>Early conduct problems<br>Use of drugs and alcohol<br>Extraversion<br>Family history of psychiatric disorder | All applied after controlling for exposure to trauma<br>Increased risk for exposure to trauma only |

# Trauma and Trauma Intensity as Risk Factors for PTSD (Table 8–7)

In the St. Louis ECA study (Helzer et al. 1987), PTSD rates were three times higher in wounded Vietnam veterans than in nonwounded combat veterans (20% versus 6.3%). PTSD symptoms were also more common in wounded than in nonwounded veterans (60% versus 43%). Among those

Vietnam-theater veterans in the NVVRS who had experienced the highest levels of exposure to extreme events in the war zone, current PTSD prevalence rates were 35.8% for men and 17.5% for women.

In the North Carolina ECA study (Winfield et al. 1990), the prevalence of PTSD in victims of sexual assault who were physically injured during the assault (14.1%) was 22 times higher than the prevalence of PTSD in non-injured victims of sexual assault (0.64%).

Pynoos and colleagues (1987) found that the frequency and severity of PTSD increased in proportion to proximity/exposure to the trauma. The modal form of PTSD for the "on playground" group (i.e., most exposed) was severe PTSD (48%); for the "in school" group (i.e., less exposed) it was moderate PTSD (50%); and the modal reaction for the "not at school" group was no PTSD (55%).

In the Card study (1987), 8 out of 10 combat-related variables were sig-

**Table 8–7.**   Contributing effect of trauma exposure to PTSD

| Study | Dose Effect of Trauma | Comments |
|---|---|---|
| Helzer et al. 1987 | Yes | Higher prevalence of PTSD in wounded combat veterans, and after controlling for preservice vulnerability |
| McFarlane 1989 | Yes at 4 months No at 11 and 29 months | Premorbid and other risk factors grew in importance for chronic PTSD |
| Card 1987 | Yes | 27% prevalence in heavy combat group, 19% prevalence in combat group as a whole |
| Shore et al. 1986a, 1986b, 1989 | Yes | 1) Increased prevalence of a group of stress-related disorders (major depressive disorder, generalized anxiety disorder, PTSD) with greater exposure to trauma, 2) premorbid risk factors only important in non-exposure group, 3) increased duration of symptoms with greater stress |
| Winfield et al. 1990 | Yes | 14% PTSD prevalence in physically injured victims of sexual assault, compared to 0.6% in noninjured victims |
| Pynoos et al. 1987 | Yes | Increased frequency/severity of PTSD in relation to proximity of sniper |
| Goldberg et al. 1990 | Yes | Increased risk as combat intensity increased; genetic contributions kept constant by nature of sample |
| NVVRS Kulka et al. 1990 | Yes | Increased frequency of current PTSD with higher combat exposure |

nificantly associated with increased risk for PTSD, as compared to only 2 out of 25 preservice and inservice variables.

The MSH study showed that the three MSH stress-related disorders (of which PTSD was one) increased in frequency with the victim's proximity to the explosion (Shore et al. 1986b). First year postdisaster onset rates of MSH stress-related disorders for males were 0.9%, 2.5%, and 11.1% in non-exposed controls, low exposure populations, and high exposure populations, respectively. Onset rates for females in these groups were 1.9%, 5.6%, and 20.9%, respectively. Unfortunately, data were unavailable for PTSD alone.

McFarlane (1989) found that trauma intensity influenced risk of PTSD only in the first few months in the full sample and remained as a persistent influence only in one subgroup of PTSD—namely, the recurrent-chronic type (McFarlane 1988b).

## Interaction of Preexisting Risk Factors With Trauma

Debate has continued as to the relative contributions of the trauma itself and the role of potential predisposing or subsequent events as determinants of PTSD. Review of recent epidemiological studies sheds some light on this issue—perhaps one of the more important issues in the study of PTSD. Several researchers hold that severe stress is not only necessary but also sufficient to account for PTSD. Clearly, without the event PTSD could not exist by definition, but are other risk factors also necessary?

McFarlane's study (1989) was unique in that he explored different risk factors in relationship to PTSD separately at 4, 11, and 29 months postdisaster. He concluded:

> The relative sizes of the contributions and the nature of the effect of premorbid characteristics and the impact of the disaster would appear to have changed with time. While extreme adversity plays a central precipitating role in the onset of post traumatic morbidity, this study raises questions about the hypothesized etiological process in PTSD, because the data at no stage demonstrated that the event had a greater formative event than did predisposing premorbid characteristics. (pp 227–228)

Interpretation of McFarlane's findings should take into account that his subjects were exposed to a brief and discrete trauma that lasted for a mean of 15 hours and was associated with minimal bereavement.

In the NVVRS (Kulka et al. 1990), the role of potential predisposing factors was examined by assessing the aggregate impact of more than 80 characteristics and experiences that predated the respondents' military service in Vietnam. Multivariate analyses indicated that, although background factors were significantly related to the current prevalence of PTSD, the current prevalence was much higher among Vietnam-theater veterans than among Vietnam-era veterans and civilian counterparts, even after background differences were taken into account. Although these findings indicated that background characteristics played a significant role in determining who developed PTSD after exposure to extreme events, they also indicated that the high current prevalence of PTSD among Vietnam veterans in 1988 cannot be explained solely on the basis of predisposing characteristics. Thus, data from the NVVRS have provided support for a conceptual model of PTSD that posits interacting roles for characteristics of both the stressor and the individual in the development of PTSD.

An important finding also arose from the MSH study (Shore et al. 1986a, 1986b). It was found that premorbid risk factors became less important as intensity of the exposure to trauma increased. When the disaster impact was most severe, the stressor overrode vulnerability factors that, at a lower level of trauma exposure, identified higher risk subgroups. This argument has been important for showing the influence of risk-group variability and different levels of stress exposure on psychiatric morbidity. Similar findings emerged in nonepidemiological studies of World War II veterans (Slater 1943; Speed et al. 1989).

A caveat mentioned by McFarlane (1989), which would appear to be applicable to all PTSD studies, indicates the importance of recall. Fire fighters who did not develop PTSD symptoms showed attrition in recall of details of a traumatic event and had on a number of occasions forgotten the fact that they had been or were injured. Failure to take recall into account might lead researchers to make spurious associations between certain event characteristics and the subsequent development of symptoms.

## Symptomatology of PTSD

The three DIS based studies have been of limited value in that their symptom algorithms were somewhat complex and in two cases required that a respondent link each specific symptom with a referent event. Although someone must make this linkage in order for the diagnosis to be made, it is not generally held that PTSD victims should be able to make such linkages, especially in cases of multiple traumas or events that occurred many years previously.

In the St. Louis study (Helzer et al. 1987), nightmares, jumpiness, and insomnia were most common (no prevalence estimates given), whereas emotional numbing and guilt were found in only 5% of the respondents. In the North Carolina ECA report (Davidson et al. 1991), intrusive imagery or acting as if in the middle of an event was present in 100% (a required item). The other most frequent symptoms were startle reaction (88%), insomnia (81%), staying on guard (79%), avoidance of reminders (65%), impaired concentration (58%), diminished interest since the event (56%), having less feeling for people (46%), and survival guilt (9%).

In the MSH PTSD group (Shore et al. 1989), the most frequently occurring symptoms were intrusive thoughts (100%), numbing of responsiveness (100%), insomnia (95%), increased startle (86%), trouble concentrating (81%), guilt/worthlessness (59%), and avoidance behavior (51%). Except for avoidance behavior and guilt, there were no apparent differences in PTSD symptoms across the stressor groups (combat, physical assault, and other trauma). In a detailed analysis of sensitivity and specificity for each symptom for the diagnosis of PTSD, McFarlane (1988a) found that intrusive imagery was highly sensitive (89%) but had a low specificity (65%). High specificity was attached to nightmares (100%), recurrent waves of feeling (97%), symptoms being activated by many triggers (97%), reduced interest (100%), increased startle (100%), survival guilt (100%), impaired concentration (100%), and avoidance of reminders (100%). An important finding was that an additional question ("Do your thoughts and feelings of the event cut across or interfere with your life?") carried a 78% sensitivity and 97% specificity for distinguishing PTSD from non-PTSD. This latter finding supported the validity of PTSD as a diagnostic category and also highlighted the central importance of intrusive symptoms at a distressing level.

Although the findings we have summarized on the prevalence of specific PTSD symptoms are of some interest, the methodological limitations of these studies must also be acknowledged. In many cases, the percentages were determined by a choice of diagnostic algorithms from the DIS data that may differ slightly from a DSM-III interview; moreover, McFarlane's series (1988a, 1988b, and 1989) is based on only nine patients with PTSD.

In the NVVRS (Kulka et al. 1990), among male Vietnam-theater veterans with current PTSD, the mean number of reexperiencing symptoms was 2.02, the mean number of avoidance symptoms was 2.80 and the mean number of arousal symptoms was 2.60. Comparable figures for female Vietnam-theater veterans with PTSD were 3.04, 2.78, and 2.04.

## Differences Between Acute and Chronic PTSD

Information regarding this issue is available from the two ECA surveys and from McFarlane's analysis. In the St. Louis study (Helzer et al. 1987), combat and physical assault were specifically associated with higher frequency of chronic PTSD. In the North Carolina ECA study (Davidson et al. 1991), combat, seeing someone hurt or killed, or being the victim of physical attack was also associated with chronicity of symptoms, whereas an unspecified category of "miscellaneous" events was associated with more self-limiting PTSD. Also in the North Carolina study, survival guilt and avoidance of reminders of the trauma were the only symptoms to be found more often in chronic PTSD. Moreover, in respect to comorbidity, social phobia and somatization disorder were significantly more frequent in individuals with chronic PTSD. Other differences noted in the North Carolina study were the lower frequency of married status and lower levels of perceived social support in chronic PTSD.

McFarlane (1989) found different sets of discriminating predictors for acute PTSD and different subtypes of chronic PTSD. The following factors were predictive of acute PTSD: avoidance of debriefings, shunning of support, and extent of property loss. For persistent chronic PTSD, neuroticism, adverse life events before the trauma, a history of treated psychiatric disorder, and avoidance of thinking through negative experiences were all viewed as significant predictors. In the case of resolved or recurrent chronic PTSD, avoidance of thinking about problems and past psychiatric history were the only two predictors. In comparing recurrent and persistent chronic PTSD, previous psychiatric history and the impact of property loss were predictive of recurrent PTSD; avoidance of negative events, neuroticism, previous psychiatric history, and adverse life events before the trauma were predictors for persistent chronic PTSD.

# Validation of PTSD: Specificity of the Stressor-PTSD Connection

If the incidence of PTSD greatly increased in contrast to other disorders among individuals exposed to an extreme event, this could be taken as indirect evidence in support of the construct validity of PTSD as a diagnostic entity. On the other hand, if the incidence or prevalence of PTSD did not particularly increase, or if a seemingly unpatterned increase in other disorders took place, then validity of the concept would be challenged. Two epidemiological data bases were available that provide information addressing this issue.

In the MSH study (Shore et al. 1989), only 3 of 14 DIS-based psychiatric disorders increased in the at-risk sample 1 year following the MSH eruption: PTSD, GAD, and single episode depression. Moreover, the combined incidence of these three disorders increased in proportion to degree of trauma exposure.

In the North Carolina ECA study, Winfield and colleagues (1990) examined the relationship between sexual assault and lifetime rates of 10 DIS-based disorders. The following disorders occurred significantly more often: major depression, alcohol abuse/dependence, drug abuse/dependence, panic disorder, PTSD and obsessive-compulsive disorder (OCD). No increases were noted in dysthymia, somatization disorder, schizophrenia/schizophreniform, or GAD. All cases of panic disorder, and 46% of OCD cases, had already emerged prior to trauma, whereas depression and alcohol and drug abuse were particularly likely to appear after trauma. Age at onset of PTSD could not be ascertained. We may conclude that both studies supported the existence of a special connection between severe trauma and increased risk of PTSD; it is noted that of all diagnoses, only PTSD and depression showed increased prevalence in association with trauma in both studies.

Depression deserves special comment because of the MSH depressed group ($n = 12$). Of these subjects, 25% exhibited avoidance of trauma symptoms, 42% had numbed responsiveness, 42% had intrusive thoughts, and 58% had hyperalertness/startle. It is possible that posttraumatic depression is as much a partial form of PTSD as it is a manifestation of depression.

# Conclusions

Lifetime and current prevalence rates of PTSD varied widely according to the diagnostic method, but these rates remained very consistent with the survey-based DIS, which generally produced lower estimates than those obtained with other methods such as the GHQ, multimethod assessments, and clinical diagnostic interview. Whatever the diagnostic method used, however, it is clear that PTSD and partial forms of PTSD combined were common in the general population, ranging from 8% to 16%, and were almost an expected and predictable response to combat (e.g., occurring in 53% of Vietnam veterans). PTSD became chronic in more than 50% of all cases and was accompanied by psychiatric comorbidity in the great majority.

Predictors of chronic morbidity have been examined by McFarlane (1988a, 1988b, 1989), who found that the role of the trauma itself was modest at best and diminished with time. Trauma's role was overshadowed by premorbid variables such as neuroticism, previous adverse life events, and previous psychiatric disorder. His finding, however, of the minimal impact of trauma itself as a predictor of chronicity should be seen in light of other studies that have indicated that more massive trauma overrides other vulnerability factors. Conversely, the NVVRS (Kulka et al. 1990) revealed that, although personal background characteristics played a significant role in PTSD prevalence, exposure to extreme events made a significant contribution to the prevalence of PTSD that was independent of the effects of personal background characteristics. These findings, which have emphasized a role for both individual vulnerability and exposure to trauma, provided support to validate the concept of PTSD as a "stress response" illness.

Psychiatric comorbidity in association with PTSD revealed that many disorders have been seen more frequently among those with PTSD. The high comorbidity with somatization disorder in the North Carolina ECA study (Davidson et al. 1991) suggested a kinship between PTSD and mechanisms of conversion and dissociation. Elevated comorbidity with many other anxiety disorders, major depression, antisocial personality disorder, and drug and alcohol abuse were also found.

Although a necessary condition, exposure to an extreme event itself is probably not sufficient to account for the diagnosis and perpetuation of PTSD, except in situations where there has been exposure to the most extreme events (e.g., abusive captivity). Nonetheless, its central importance as a necessary feature has been substantiated by epidemiological surveys. Thus, PTSD rates were greater than the base rate in individuals selected for exposure to a specific trauma and continued to increase as the trauma was more intense (e.g., wounded versus nonwounded combat veterans, degree of exposure to war zone stress, physically injured versus nonphysically injured victims of sexual assault, people living closer to the MSH eruption versus those who lived farther away, or children in the playground versus those in the building versus those not at school during a sniper attack). A dose-effect relationship would thus appear to exist for PTSD with respect to the trauma exposure (see Chapter 3 by March).

In two epidemiological studies (Shore et al. 1989; Winfield et al. 1990) that examined morbidity following trauma, only PTSD and depression were noted to increase in both studies. This finding lends good support to the view that extreme stress is not merely a nonspecific trigger for a variety of illnesses. Rather, the data support the concept that some events are unusually distressing in a way that is linked specifically with PTSD symptoms.

The MSH results also suggested that other psychiatric conditions (i.e., major depression and GAD) included symptoms of PTSD, thus indicating the possibility that they may have been subclinical forms of PTSD enmeshed with, or determining the expression of, another disorder. We would raise for consideration the possibility that there exists a subtype of depression following trauma ("posttraumatic depression") that differs in important ways from clinical major depression of nontraumatic type. A person might thus experience such a posttraumatic depressive reaction, without meeting diagnostic criteria for PTSD.

As further data become available to support the possibility that individuals experience a variety of posttraumatic responses (e.g., depression, anxiety, dissociative reaction), the case may become stronger for considering a separate category of disorders that develop following traumatic stress. Such an approach would also be compatible with the position taken by the *International Classification of Diseases, 10th Revision* (ICD-10).

# References

American Psychiatric Association: Diagnostic and Statistical Manual of Mental Disorders, 3rd Edition. Washington, DC, American Psychiatric Association, 1980

American Psychiatric Association: Diagnostic and Statistical Manual of Mental Disorders, 3rd Edition, Revised. Washington, DC, American Psychiatric Association, 1987

Breslau N, Davis GC, Andreski P: Traumatic events and post traumatic stress disorder in an urban population of young adults. Arch Gen Psychiatry 48:216–222, 1991

Card JJ: Epidemiology of PTSD in a national cohort of Vietnam veterans. J Clin Psychol 43:6–17, 1987

Centers for Disease Control: Health status of Vietnam veterans: psychosocial characteristics. JAMA 259:2701–2707, 1988

Davidson JRT, Hughes D, Blazer D, et al: Post traumatic stress disorder in the community: an epidemiological study. Psychol Med 21:1–9, 1991

Goldberg DP: The Detection of Psychiatric Illness by Questionnaire. London, Oxford University Press, 1972

Goldberg J, True WR, Eisen SA, et al: A twin study of the effects of the Vietnam war on post traumatic stress disorder. JAMA 263:1227–1232, 1990

Hathaway SR, McKinley JC: Minnesota Multiphasic Personality Inventory—2. Minneapolis, MN, University of Minnesota, 1989

Helzer JE, Robins LN, McEvoy L: Post traumatic stress disorder in the general population. New Engl J Med 317:1630–1634, 1987

Horowitz M, Wilner N, Alvarez W: Impact of Event Scale: a measure of subjective stress. Psychosom Med 41:209–218, 1979

Keane TM, Wolfe J: Comorbidity in post traumatic stress disorder: an analysis of community and clinical studies. Journal of Applied Social Psychology 20:1776–1788, 1990

Keane TM, Malloy PF, Fairbank JA: Empirical development of an MMPI subscale for the assessment of combat-related posttraumatic stress disorder. J Consult Clin Psychol 52:888–891, 1984

Keane TM, Caddell JM, Taylor KL: Mississippi Scale for Combat-Related Post Traumatic Stress Disorder: three studies in reliability and validity. J Consult Clin Psychol 56:85–90, 1988

Kulka RA, Schlenger WE: Survey research and field designs for the study of posttraumatic stress disorder, in International Handbook of Traumatic Stress Syndromes. Edited by Wilson J, Raphael B. New York, Plenum (in press)

Kulka RA, Schlenger WE, Fairbank JA, et al: Trauma and the Vietnam War Generation. New York, Brunner/Mazel, 1990

Kulka R, Schlenger WE, Fairbank JA, et al: Assessment of PTSD in the community: prospects and pitfalls from recent studies of Vietnam veterans. Psychological Assessment: A Journal of Consulting and Clinical Psychology (in press)

Last JM: A Dictionary of Epidemiology. New York, Oxford University Press, 1983

Mai FM, Merskey H: Briquet's treatise on hysteria: synopsis and commentary. Arch Gen Psychiatry 37:1401–1405, 1980

McFarlane AC: The phenomenology of post traumatic stress disorders following a natural disaster. J Nerv Ment Dis 176:22–29, 1988a

McFarlane AC: The longitudinal course of post traumatic morbidity. J Nerv Ment Dis 176:30–39, 1988b

McFarlane AC: The aetiology of post traumatic morbidity: predisposing, precipitating and perpetuating factors. Br J Psychiatry 154:221–228, 1989

Pynoos RS, Frederick C, Nader K, et al; Life threat and post traumatic stress in school-age children. Arch Gen Psychiatry 12:1057–1063, 1987

Robins LN, Helzer JE, Croughan JL, et al: NIMH Diagnostic Interview Schedule: Version III (DHHS Publ No ADM-T-42-3 [5-8] [8-81]). Rockville, MD, National Institute of Mental Health, Public Health Service, 1981

Shore JH: The Mt. St. Helen's stress response syndrome, in Disaster Stress Studies: New Methods and Findings. Edited by Shore JH. Washington, DC, American Psychiatric Press, 1986, pp 78–97

Shore JH, Tatum E, Vollmer WM: Evaluation of mental health effects of disaster: Mt. St. Helen's eruption. Am J Public Health 76:76–83, 1986a

Shore JH, Tatum E, Vollmer WM: Psychiatric reactions to disaster: the Mt. St. Helen's experience. Am J Psychiatry 143:590–595, 1986b

Shore JH, Vollmer WM, Tatum EL: Community patterns of post traumatic stress disorders. J Nerv Ment Dis 177:681–685, 1989

Slater E: The neurotic constitution. J Neurol Psychiatry 6:1–6, 1943

Snow BR, Stellman JM, Stellman SD, et al: Post-traumatic stress disorder among American Legionnaires in relation to combat experience in Vietnam: associated and contributory factors. Environ Res 47:175–192, 1988

Speed N, Engdahl B, Schwartz J, et al: Post traumatic stress disorder as a consequence of the POW experience. J Nerv Ment Dis 177:147–153, 1989

Spitzer RL, Williams JB, Gibbon M: Structured Clinical Interview for DSM-III-R, Version NP-V. New York, Biometrics Research Department. New York State Psychiatric Institute, 1987

Weiss DS, Horowitz MJ, Wilner N: The Stress Response Rating Scale: a clinician's measure for rating the response to serious life events. Br J Clin Psychol 23:202–215, 1984

Weissman MM, Myers JK, Ross CE (eds): Community Surveys of Psychiatric Disorders. New Brunswick, NJ, Rutgers University Press, 1986

Winfield I, George LK, Swartz M, et al: Sexual assault and psychiatric disorders among women in a community population. Am J Psychiatry 147:335–341, 1990

◆

# Section IV:

# Classification of Posttraumatic Stress Disorder

◆

# ◆ 9 ◆ Biological Findings in Posttraumatic Stress Disorder: Implications for DSM-IV Classification

Roger K. Pitman, M.D.

***Summary*** **B**iological findings in posttraumatic stress disorder (PTSD) are reviewed from the standpoint of two questions: 1) How can they can guide us in the proper classification of PTSD? and 2) Do they suggest the need for any revision of diagnostic criteria? The author groups PTSD symptomatology into tonic (enduring) and phasic (intermittent) features and reviews the literature on each. These are then grouped into autonomic, neuroregulatory, endocrinological, sleep, treatment outcome studies, and biological models of PTSD. A hierarchical approach to method of classification is given and then applied to PTSD. A recommendation is made for classifying PTSD by etiology, and the placement of certain symptoms is addressed.

## Statement of the Issue

The issues to be addressed in this review are how biological findings in PTSD research to date can inform the proper location of this disorder in psychiatric classification, as exemplified by DSM-IV, and appropriate revisions of diagnostic criteria for the disorder.

## Methods

A literature search was undertaken on the biology of PTSD, covering the period 1980–1989, and other unpublished sources were also identified for inclusion in this review.

# Results

As currently defined, PTSD consists of a combination of tonic and phasic features. The "tonic" features are those that the patient manifests all or most of the time and that constitute a part of his or her baseline mental functioning. The "phasic" features are only manifest from time to time, especially when they are evoked by a salient environmental event. The DSM-III-R criteria (American Psychiatric Association 1987) divide PTSD symptoms into three major categories: intrusion, avoidance (or numbing), and arousal. Although patients may complain of the frequency and intensity of their nightmares, flashbacks, and intrusive recollections, intrusion symptoms are phasic rather than tonic. In contrast to the intrusion symptoms, the avoidance symptoms of PTSD are tonic. Diminished interest, numbing, and estrangement characterize the PTSD patient's baseline functioning. Avoidance of reminders of the traumatic event derives from the painful phasic recollections that the reminders trigger. The third category of PTSD symptom (i.e., arousal) comprises a mixture of tonic and phasic symptoms. Examples of tonic arousal symptoms include insomnia and hypervigilance; examples of phasic arousal symptoms include exaggerated startle response and "physiological reactivity upon exposure to events that symbolize or resemble an aspect of the traumatic event." In this review, I accordingly divide the biological PTSD findings into tonic and phasic aspects.

## Tonic Aspects of PTSD

Biological studies of the tonic aspects of PTSD have included a variety of autonomic, neuroregulatory, and endocrinological dependent variables measured in a baseline or resting condition.

### Autonomic Studies

Most recent studies designed to evaluate phasic autonomic responses (Blanchard et al. 1982, 1986; Malloy et al. 1983; Pitman et al. 1987) have found baseline heart rate (HR) and blood pressure (BP) elevations in PTSD compared to various control subjects prior to the presentation of the experimental stimuli. My colleagues and I found baseline HR differences between PTSD subjects and non-PTSD anxiety disorder control subjects (Pitman et al. 1990a). However, there is some question as to whether subjects in these experiments can be considered to be in a truly tonic state, or whether they are under the influence of anticipating the coming experiment, in which case the elevations could represent phasic activity. Davidson and Baum (1986) reported higher mean HR and systolic and diastolic BP in (nondiagnosed) stressed individuals living within 5 miles of a damaged nuclear power station, compared to control subjects living 80 miles away.

Although it is likely that this increased tonic sympathetic activity represents an acquired phenomenon in PTSD, almost no data are available on PTSD individuals regarding their autonomic state prior to the trauma. This would be required to demonstrate conclusively that the hyperactivity is the result of the traumatic event. However, in unpublished work, my colleagues and I have examined the pre-Vietnam military induction pulse rates and BPs of large samples of veterans who went on to develop PTSD after combat and of veterans who did not develop PTSD. They found that the mean pre-Vietnam pulse rate of the PTSD veterans was actually 2.5 beats per minute *lower* than the control subjects (nonsignificant difference), and the mean systolic and diastolic BPs of the two groups were nearly identical, supporting the absence of sympathetic hyperactivity in the PTSD subjects prior to their traumatic combat events.

### Neuroregulatory Studies

Davidson and Baum (1986) also found elevated norepinephrine excretions in the same stressed residents living within 5 miles of the damaged nuclear power station cited previously. Kosten and colleagues (1987) found increased 24-hour norepinephrine and epinephrine excretions in diagnosed Vietnam veteran PTSD inpatients when compared to control inpatients with non-PTSD mental disorders. However, Orr and I (Pitman and Orr 1990) were unable to replicate this findings using non-PTSD combat veteran control subjects.

Interesting indirect evidence for tonic sympathetic hyperactivity in PTSD is provided by studies of peripheral adrenergic receptor systems. Perry and associates (1987, 1990) reported reduced in vitro total $\alpha$-2-adrenergic receptor binding sites, and an increased $\alpha$-2-(L)/$\alpha$-2-(H) affinity state ratio, in the platelets of Vietnam veteran subjects with PTSD compared to control subjects without PTSD. Lerer and colleagues (1987b) found lower in vitro basal and stimulated platelet and lymphocyte $\beta$-adrenergic receptor-mediated cyclic adenosine 3′,5′-monophosphate (cAMP) signal transduction in Israeli PTSD subjects compared to control subjects without PTSD. These receptor changes are consistent with downregulation resulting from exposure to elevated levels of circulating catecholamines.

Finally, Davidson and colleagues (1985) reported lower platelet mono-amine oxidase (MAO) activity, which may be a risk factor for psychopathology, in PTSD veterans compared to control subjects. The observed group differences, however, were mainly due to low MAO activity in the alcoholic subgroup of PTSD subjects, confounding interpretation of the results.

### Endocrinological Studies

Results of research into the classic endocrinological manifestation of the stress response, viz. hyperactivity of the hypothalamic-pituitary-adrenal-cortical (HYPAC) axis, in PTSD have been conflicting. Mason and colleagues (1986) actually found significantly *decreased* 24-hour urinary free cortisol (UFC) excretion in PTSD inpatients compared to inpatients with other diagnoses. Orr and I, however, reported the opposite finding of significantly (though modestly) *increased* 24-hour UFC excretion in PTSD, in comparison to non-PTSD combat veterans (Pitman and Orr 1990). Davidson and Baum (1986) also found elevated cortisol excretions in their stressed residents living near the damaged nuclear power station. Smith and colleagues (1989) found severity of PTSD symptoms in combat veterans to correlate directly with basal plasma cortisol level. The primary finding reported by these authors was diminished pituitary secretion of adrenocorticotropic hormone (ACTH) in response to in vivo corticotropin releasing hormone (CRH) challenge. This indirectly tends to support high circulating cortisol in PTSD. However, an alternate explanation suggested by Smith and colleagues is either pituitary depletion or desensitization due to persistent elevation of endogenous CRH, supporting the possibility of HYPAC axis overactivity at the level of the hypothalamus.

An abnormal dexamethasone suppression test (DST) appears to be rare in PTSD (Kudler et al. 1987). Halbreich and colleagues (1988) found that even PTSD patients with comorbid symptomatic major depression did not have abnormal DSTs, as opposed to many non-PTSD cases of major depression, and concluded that the depression found in PTSD is biologically different. Smith and colleagues (1989) have observed that the HYPAC axis abnormalities in PTSD—abnormal CRH test, normal DST, and normal urinary cortisol excretion (although findings are divergent in this last regard)—most resemble those found in patients with panic disorder.

### Sleep Studies

Results of sleep studies in PTSD are consistent with chronically disturbed sleep associated with excessive arousal. Kaminer and Lavie (1988) found that poorly adjusted Jewish survivors of the Holocaust in World War II (presumably with PTSD) had longer sleep latencies, more awakenings, less sleep time, and lower sleep efficiency than well-adjusted survivors and control subjects. The same pattern of disturbed sleep was found by van Kammen and colleagues (1990) in American World War II prisoners of war (POWs) with PTSD. Such findings more than 40 years after the trauma dramatically illustrate the tenacity of the arousal disturbance in PTSD. Kinney and Kramer (1985) also found PTSD patients to be more reactive to nonspecific auditory stimuli experimentally presented during sleep. Studies of PTSD have not found decreased rapid eye movement (REM) latency or increased REM activity, the hallmarks of the sleep disturbance in endogenous depression. The findings in PTSD subjects are not dissimilar to findings in panic disorder, in which sleep latency is increased and sleep time and efficiency are decreased but REM latency is not consistently shortened (Mellman and Uhde 1989).

## Phasic Aspects of PTSD

Biological studies of the phasic aspects of PTSD are more challenging, because in addition to whatever dependent variables are employed (unless one is prepared to wait for phasic changes to occur spontaneously), one or more independent stimulus variables are required to elicit them. Phasic studies may be considered biological if either the independent or dependent variables are biological. With the notable exception of research employing a biochemical stimulus (sodium lactate) in the elicitation of flashbacks and panic anxiety in PTSD (Rainey et al. 1987), it is the dependent variables that have been biological in phasic PTSD studies.

A useful working framework within which to interpret these studies is that of classical conditioning. Within this framework, the traumatic event is seen to serve as an unconditioned stimulus (UCS). Subsequently, stimuli associated with or resembling the traumatic event come to act as conditioned stimuli (CSs) to elicit conditioned responses (CRs) in the form of PTSD symptoms or measurable physiological responses.

### Autonomic Studies

There is now a robust literature documenting phasic autonomic hyperresponsivity to combat-related audiovisual stimuli in PTSD compared to various groups of comparison subjects, including nonveterans (Blanchard et al. 1982), mentally healthy combat veterans (Blanchard et al. 1986; Malloy et al. 1983; Pallmeyer et al. 1986) and non-PTSD psychiatric patients (Malloy et al. 1983; Pallmeyer et al. 1986). My colleagues and I (Pitman et al. 1987) have also found PTSD veterans to be autonomically (and musculoskeletally) hyperresponsive to individualized imagery of their combat experiences, but not to imagery of other past stressful events not forming the basis for their PTSD symptoms. Recently, we found that combat veterans with non-PTSD anxiety disorders were not hyperresponsive to their combat imagery (Pitman et al. 1990a). These findings indicate that PTSD represents more than the coincidental occurrence of stressful events in anxiety-prone individuals. In both studies, we found that PTSD subjects' self-reported anger and sadness responses were as great as their fear responses, indicating that the emotional disturbance in PTSD is not limited to anxiety. Across psychophysiological studies to date, approximately one-third of PTSD subjects have been found to be physiological nonresponders. These studies have been unable to definitively characterize what makes these veterans different. On the other hand, there has been a near-zero rate of hyperresponders among non-PTSD control subjects. These findings indicate a higher specificity than sensitivity for the psychophysiological method in the detection of interview-diagnosed cases of PTSD.

### Neuroregulatory and Endocrinological Studies

McFall and colleagues (1990) found that PTSD subjects had greater arterialized plasma epinephrine, as well as pulse and BP, responses to a combat film than a mixed group of control subjects. The authors cite these results as supporting the autonomic conditioning theory of PTSD.

A recent pilot study (Pitman et al. 1990b; van der Kolk et al. 1989) found that PTSD subjects, but not healthy combat control subjects, showed a naloxone-reversible decrease in pain sensibility after viewing a combat videotape. These results are consistent with the development of phasic opioid-mediated stress-induced analgesia (SIA) in PTSD. SIA is a well-documented manifestation of the stress response in animals observed in conditions of learned helplessness and conditioned fear.

All the above findings have involved the responses of PTSD veterans to combat-related (conditioned) stimuli. There has also been recent work regarding responses to nonspecific stressful stimuli in PTSD as well. Hamner and Hitri (1989) found greater plasma β-endorphin responses to exercise in PTSD Vietnam veterans compared to noncombat veterans who were control subjects. Although Ornitz and Pynoos (1989) found the unwarned blink reflex startle responses to bursts of white noise of PTSD children to be (surprisingly) smaller than those of non-PTSD children, there was also some evidence supporting a loss of inhibitory modulation of the startle response in the PTSD children, consistent with experimental findings in animal stress research.

### Lactate-Induced Panic

Rainey and colleagues (1987) studied the effect of intravenous double-blind sodium lactate, isoproterenol, or dextrose infusion in a group of seven PTSD Vietnam veterans, all of whom had a history of flashbacks and six of whom had comorbid panic disorder. All seven patients had flashbacks with lactate, followed in six by panic anxiety. Three of the lactate flashbacks were to events that had occurred in hospitals, suggesting an influence of hospital-related CSs at the time of the infusion upon the material produced in the flashbacks. It is also plausible that sodium lactate induces physiological changes similar to physiological changes that had occurred at the time of the traumatic event and that, through an interoceptive mechanism, these physiological changes act as CSs to elicit a CR in the form of reexperiencing of the event as a flashback. An important limitation of this research is that subjects without flashbacks and/or panic disorder, who constitute a substantial portion (and possibly the majority) of PTSD subjects, were not studied, raising a question as to the applicability of the findings to PTSD in general.

## Pharmacological Aspects of PTSD

The pharmacology of PTSD has been reviewed in detail elsewhere (Davidson et al. 1990a, 1990b; Friedman 1988; van der Kolk 1987) and will not be treated at length here, because the nosological implications at this time are limited. A wide range of agents have been reported to be of benefit in open clinical trials. Worth noting in passing are the potential therapeutic effects of two classes of agents: the anticonvulsant carbamazepine (Lipper et al. 1986; Wolf et al. 1988), because this provides potential support for the kindling hypothesis of PTSD (see next section); and sympathetic agents such as the β-adrenergic blocker propranolol and the α-2-adrenergic agonist clonidine (Kolb et al. 1984), because this supports the importance of sympathetic arousal in the disorder.

A pharmacotherapeutic effect has only been demonstrated in controlled double-blind studies for antidepressants (Davidson et al. 1990a; Frank et al. 1988). However, the magnitude of the therapeutic effect may be only modest (Davidson et al. 1990a; Lerer et al. 1987a; Shestatzky et al. 1988). Interestingly, the effect seems to favor the specific intrusive PTSD symptoms, rather than the more generalized numbing and avoidance systems (Davidson et al. 1990a; Frank et al. 1988), which bear at least a superficially closer resemblance to the symptoms of depression.

## Biological Models of PTSD

Several theoretical biological models deriving from basic research have been advanced to account for PTSD and are listed below.

**Inescapable shock.**    Van der Kolk and colleagues (1985) argued that the sequelae of inescapable shock in animals, which include learned helplessness and SIA, show parallels to the sequelae of psychic trauma in humans. The finding of an analgesic response to a combat stimulus in PTSD veterans reviewed previously offers some support for this model.

**Kindling.**    Several authors (Friedman 1988; Lipper et al. 1986; van der Kolk and Greenberg 1987) have observed that the experimental animal phenomenon of kindling, in which cumulative electrical or pharmacological stimulation may sensitize limbic neuronal circuits and lower neuronal firing thresholds, may be a useful model for the effect on the brain of exposure and reexposure to traumatic stimuli. As noted previously, reports of a therapeutic effect in PTSD of the antikindling drug carbamazepine offer some support for this model.

**Superconditioning.** Studies in animals have shown that neurohormones/neuroregulators may influence the strength of CRs, and the consolidation of memory traces, in experimental animals. Pitman (1988, 1989) has hypothesized that neurohormones/neuroregulators mobilized at the time of a traumatic event may mediate an overconsolidation of the memory trace of the event, a process he has termed "superconditioning."

**Noradrenergic dysregulation.** Krystal and colleagues (1989) have argued that the noradrenergic locus coeruleus meets the criteria for a brain "trauma center," and that activation of this center, which may occur as a learned traumatic response, elicits fear behaviors similar to the alarmlike symptoms of PTSD.

**Neuropsychological sensitization.** Kolb (1987, 1988) has postulated that excessive stimulation, as may occur in trauma, leads to synaptic changes related to neurophysiological sensitization, depression of synaptic processes underlying habituation and discriminative perception (which Kolb holds to be a central phenomenon in PTSD), and even potential neuronal death.

**Stress-induced sensitization to subsequent stressors.** Antelman (1988) has noted that a number of onetime or repeated stressful manipulations may sensitize experimental animals to the effects of later lesser stressors. He has suggested that this may serve as a useful model of the poor tolerance of PTSD subjects to everyday stress.

# Discussion

## Analogy With Medical Disorders

Medical illnesses may be classified on the basis of any of the following: 1) symptomatology, 2) anatomical change, 3) pathogenesis, or 4) etiology. The historical evolution of medical diagnosis shows that this sequence constitutes a hierarchy of desirability in the nosology of disorders. Medical disorders have only been classified on the basis of their symptoms when inadequate evidence has been available concerning their other aspects. The history of medicine is replete with examples of symptomatic classifications yielding to an understanding of anatomy, pathogenesis, or etiology. For example, it was learned long ago that dropsy or edema (i.e., pathological accumulation of fluid) could arise from disturbance in a number of different organ systems, including the liver, kidneys, heart, and peripheral veins. Whether edema is based on underlying hepatic, renal, cardiac, or venous pathology has gravely different implications for both its prognosis and treatment. In our present state of knowledge, no physician would make a diagnosis of edema. It is a symptom only.

Moving up the hierarchy, classification by either anatomical lesion or pathogenesis is considered undesirable when etiology becomes known. An example is tuberculosis. Prior to the identification of the tubercle bacillus as the causal agent in this disorder, much information was available about underlying tuberculous pathological changes in the lungs, and how these changes resulted in pulmonary insufficiency and other symptoms. However, today tuberculosis is understood, and classified, not as a granulomatous structural disorder, but as an infectious disease.

## Current Classification of PTSD

The current classification of PTSD in DSM-III (American Psychiatric Association 1980) and DSM-III-R represents a curious hybrid. These manuals were avowedly written on the basis of a *symptomatic* classification of mental disorders, because of the opinion that insufficient information was available regarding their etiology or even pathogenesis. PTSD is currently classified among the anxiety disorders presumably because it is accompanied by the concomitants of anxiety (e.g., insomnia, exaggerated startle response, and difficulty concentrating). Peculiarly, it is possible for a patient to qualify for the PTSD diagnosis without any symptomatic anxiety (also the case for obsessive-compulsive disorder). The current anxiety disorder category in fact represents a carryover from Freudian theory, which posited a central role for anxiety in the *pathogenesis* of neurotic disorders.

From yet another standpoint, the specification in DSM-III and DSM-III-R of an extreme traumatic event as a necessary criterion for the disorder has unstated implications for PTSD's *etiology*. In other words, PTSD's current nosological status represents an amalgam of symptomatic, pathogenetic, and etiological classification.

## The Etiology of PTSD

Given the desirability of classifying disorders according to etiology whenever possible, the first question to be asked of the biological findings in PTSD summarized previously is: Do they support a causal role for a traumatic event in PTSD? The answer to this question appears to be that they do. If the biological findings in PTSD to date are not profound, they at least appear to be coherent. The best documented biological finding in PTSD is physiological hyperresponsivity to stimuli resembling the original traumatic event, which by definition cannot occur unless such an event occurred to begin with. As reviewed previously, psychophysiological studies have demonstrated a specific link between traumatic event and subsequent PTSD symptomatology. Hyperresponsivity to stimuli resembling past stressful events does not appear to be shared by other non-PTSD anxiety disorders.

The other major biological finding in PTSD is tonic hyperactivity of the sympathetic nervous system, manifest in physiological, neurological, endocrinological, and sleep studies. Although this has not been demonstrated in studies to date, in all likelihood the hyperaroused state of PTSD has its onset with the traumatic event(s) as well; for example, it is difficult to imagine that the World War II Holocaust survivors and POWs cited previously suffered from their sleep disturbances prior to their extreme traumatic events.

Because applicability of any of the animal models listed previously to human PTSD has not been established, they should not be afforded undue weight in psychiatric nosological determinations. However, an important element common to all of them is that they postulate an initially intact organism prior to the occurrence of the traumatic stressor. Therefore our current understanding of basic psychobiology allows for several alternate possible explanations of how an external traumatic event may cause a phenomenon such as PTSD.

## The Pathogenesis of PTSD

The data reviewed here support a role for classical conditioning in the pathogenesis PTSD, although the biological mechanisms whereby this occurs can only be the subject of speculation at this time. The relevance of so-called two-factor learning theory, involving classical conditioning followed by operant conditioning, to PTSD intrusion and avoidance symptoms respectively, has been cited as supportive of a central role for anxiety in the disorder. However, there does not appear to be any reason why other unpleasant emotions (e.g., sadness, anger, and guilt) cannot either be classically conditioned or form the basis of subsequent avoidance behavior. In other words, although two-factor conditioning is sometimes treated as synonymous with the mechanism of anxiety, it may be a broader model of emotion that subsumes but is not limited to anxiety.

Rainey and colleagues' (1987) lactate challenge study does support the role of anxiety in PTSD's pathogenesis. However, this single revealing experiment did not incorporate a representative sample of PTSD subjects, but instead selected the subject most likely to demonstrate the phenomenon. Furthermore, the findings do not imply a common *etiology* of panic disorder and PTSD. Pure panic disorder patients rarely, if ever, have flashbacks during panic attacks. The origin of the attacks in panic disorder is typically obscure, whereas in PTSD it is evident in the original traumatic event.

Dissociation may be viewed as either a pathogenetic mechanism or a symptom. Insofar as flashbacks are dissociative symptoms, their precipitation by lactate infusion suggests a link between the induction of panic anxiety and the production of dissociation. Otherwise, the available biological data in PTSD are rather mute concerning the appropriateness of using dissociation as a basis for the disorder's classification.

### The Biological "Symptomatology" of PTSD

The frequently observed comorbidity of PTSD and depression, and the therapeutic benefit of antidepressant medications in PTSD, might be construed to suggest a homologous relationship between PTSD and depression. However, their biological profiles diverge significantly. The major biological findings in endogenous depression (viz., escape from dexamethasone suppression and decreased REM-sleep latency) have been found to be absent in PTSD. It may be recalled that the so-called "antidepressants" are equally effective antipanic medications. Indeed, a better case may be made for similarity between the biological profiles of PTSD and panic disorder. As reviewed above, the two disorders appears to share common sleep and endocrinological findings.

In the occurrence of phasic autonomic hyperresponsivity to specific stimuli, PTSD resembles the simple phobias and phobic types of obsessive-compulsive disorder, but not agoraphobia (panic disorder) or generalized anxiety disorder, where such specific responses have been found to be absent (Cook et al. 1988; Lang 1985). However, with regard to tonic autonomic hyperactivity, the opposite relationship of PTSD to its anxiety disorder neighbors appears to exist. Specifically, patients with simple phobias typically lack tonic hyperarousal, whereas patients with generalized anxiety disorder (GAD) and panic disorder possess it. In short, PTSD appears to represent a uniquely unfortunate combination of the specific stimulus-induced phasic physiological hyperresponsivity of the phobic disorders and the tonic physiological hyperarousal of the panic and generalized anxiety disorders.

# Recommendations

## Implications for Classification of PTSD

The available biological data in PTSD support its independent and separate etiological classification as a posttraumatic disorder. Given the preference for medical classification by etiology whenever it can be achieved, it is the position here that this is the most appropriate classification of PTSD in DSM-IV. Classification by etiology would have the virtue of emphasizing the primary importance of prevention of traumatic events in public health considerations. Were there to be compelling arguments against an etiological classification (which I do not think there are), a pathogenetically or symptomatically based classification of PTSD as an anxiety disorder might be regarded as acceptable from the standpoint of the biological data reviewed in this chapter.

In the absence of endocrinological documentation of PTSD as a "stress" disorder, the appropriateness of continuing to incorporate this vague and hackneyed term in the disorder's appellation deserves reexamination. "Posttraumatic mental disorder" would have the virtue of simplicity. Alternately, substitution of one of the better documented features (e.g., "reexperiencing" or "arousal") might be considered. I favor "posttraumatic reexperiencing disorder," with reexperiencing understood to include physiological as well as psychological manifestations.

## Implications for the Diagnostic Criteria of PTSD

Another question is what the available biological data dictate as to proper defining characteristics of PTSD. The overall conclusion from this review is that the current DSM-III-R criteria appear to be more or less appropriate. Requiring Criterion A (i.e., the traumatic event) as necessary to the diagnosis is supported by the biological data, which as argued here justify its specifications as the disorder's cause. A prominent place for physiological hyperresponsivity to events resembling the traumatic event is also justified by the research record. In DSM-III-R, this is neither a necessary nor sufficient criterion. Because physiological nonresponsivity in the laboratory is not uncommon in subjects diagnosed as PTSD on interview, it may not yet be time to require physiological hyperresponsivity as a necessary criterion. On the hand, because physiological hyperresponsivity is rare among non-PTSD subjects, this criterion might be considered for status as sufficient for at least one necessary element in the PTSD diagnosis. Baseline sympathetic nervous system activity currently appears in DSM-III-R in the form of the arousal symptoms. Whereas no one would argue that resting hyperarousal should be sufficient to make the PTSD diagnosis, the available biological data appear to justify its status as necessary.

# References

American Psychiatric Association: Diagnostic and Statistical Manual of Mental Disorders, 3rd Edition. Washington, DC, American Psychiatric Association, 1980

American Psychiatric Association: Diagnostic and Statistical Manual of Mental Disorders, 3rd Edition, Revised. Washington, DC, American Psychiatric Association, 1987

Antelman SM: Stressor-induced sensitization to subsequent stressor: an animal model of posttraumatic stress disorder. Paper presented at the Annual Meeting of the American College of Neuropsychopharmacology, San Juan, Puerto Rico, December 16, 1988

Blanchard EB, Mold LC, Pallmeyer TP, et al: A psychophysiological study of post traumatic stress disorder in Vietnam veterans. Psychiatr Q 54:220–229, 1982

Blanchard BE, Kolb LC, Gerardi RJ, et al: Cardiac response to relevant stimuli as an adjunctive tool for diagnosing post-traumatic stress disorder in Vietnam veterans. Behavior Therapy 17:592–606, 1986

Cook EW, Melamed BG, Cuthbert BN, et al: Emotional imagery and the differential diagnosis of anxiety. J Consult Clin Psychol 56:734–740, 1988

Davidson LM, Baum A: Chronic stress and posttraumatic stress disorders. J Consult Clin Psychol 54:303–308, 1986

Davidson JRT, Lipper S, Kilts CD, et al: Platelet MAO activity in posttraumatic stress disorder. Am J Psychiatry 142:1341–1343, 1985

Davidson JRT, Kudler HS, Smith RD, et al: Amitriptyline and placebo in the treatment of posttraumatic stress disorder: a controlled trial. Arch Gen Psychiatry 47:259–266, 1990a

Davidson JRT, Kudler HS, Smith RD: Assessment and pharmacotherapy of post traumatic stress disorder, in Biological Assessment and Treatment of Post Traumatic Stress Disorder. Edited by Giller EL. Washington, DC, American Psychiatric Press, 1990b, pp 203–232

Frank JB, Kosten TR, Giller EL, et al: A randomized clinical trial of phenelzine and imipramine for posttraumatic stress disorder. Am J Psychiatry 145:1289–1291, 1988

Friedman MJ: Toward rational pharmacotherapy for posttraumatic stress disorder: an interim report. Am J Psychiatry 145:281–285, 1988

Halbreich U, Olympia J, Glogowski J, et al; The importance of past psychological trauma and pathophysiological process as determinants of current biological abnormalities. Arch Gen Psychiatry 45:293–294, 1988

Hamner MB, Hitri A: Plasma ß-endorphin in PTSD. Paper presented at the annual meeting of the American Psychiatric Association, San Francisco, CA, May 8, 1989

Kaminer H, Lavie P: Dreaming and long term adjustment to severe trauma. Sleep Research 18:146, 1988

Kinney L, Kramer M: Sleep and sleep responsivity in disturbed dreamers. Sleep Research 14:178, 1985

Kolb LC: A neuropsychological hypothesis explaining posttraumatic stress disorder. Am J Psychiatry 144:989–995, 1987

Kolb LC: A critical survey of hypotheses regarding post-traumatic stress disorders in light of recent research findings. Journal of Traumatic Stress 1:291–304, 1988

Kolb LC, Burris BC, Griffiths S: Propranolol and clonidine in the treatment of post traumatic stress disorders of war, in Post Traumatic Stress Disorders: Psychological and Biological Sequelae. Edited by van der Kolk BA. Washington, DC, American Psychiatric Press, 1984, pp 97–107

Kosten TR, Mason JW, Giller EL, et al: Sustained urinary norepinephrine and epinephrine elevation in post-traumatic stress disorder. Psychoneuroendocrinology 12:13-20, 1987

Krystal JH, Kosten TR, Southwick S, et al: Neurobiological aspects of PTSD: review of clinical and preclinical studies. Behavior Therapy 20:177–198, 1989

Kudler H, Davidson J, Meador K, et al: The DST and posttraumatic stress disorder. Am J Psychiatry 144:1068–1071, 1987

Lang PJ: The cognitive psychophysiology of emotion: fear and anxiety, in Anxiety and the Anxiety Disorders. Edited by Tuma AH, Maser J. Hillsdale, NJ, Lawrence Erlbaum Associates, 1985, pp 131–170

Lerer B, Bleich A, Kotler M, et al: Posttraumatic stress disorder in Israeli combat veterans: effect of phenelzine treatment. Arch Gen Psychiatry 44:976–981, 1987a

Lerer B, Ebstein RP, Shestatsky M, et al: Cyclic AMP signal transduction in posttraumatic stress disorder. Am J Psychiatry 144:1324–1327, 1987b

Lipper S, Davidson JRT, Grady TA, et al: Preliminary study of carbamazepine in post-traumatic stress disorder. Psychosomatics 27:849–854, 1986

Malloy PF, Fairbank JA, Keane TM: Validation of a multimethod assessment of posttraumatic stress disorders in Vietnam veterans. J Consult Clin Psychol 51:488–494, 1983

Mason JW, Giller EL, Kosten TR, et al: Urinary free-cortisol levels in posttraumatic stress disorder patients. J Nerv Ment Dis 174:145–149, 1986

McFall ME, Murburg MM, Ko GN, et al: Autonomic responses to stress in Vietnam combat veterans with post-traumatic stress disorder. Biol Psychiatry 27:1165–1175, 1990

Mellman TA, Uhde TW. Electroencephalographic sleep in panic disorder. Arch Gen Psychiatry 46:178–184, 1989

Ornitz EM, Pynoos RS: Startle modulation in children with posttraumatic stress disorder. Am J Psychiatry 146:866–870, 1989

Pallmeyer TP, Blanchard EB, Kolb LC: The psychophysiology of combat-induced post-traumatic stress disorder in Vietnam veterans. Behav Res Ther 24:645–652, 1986

Perry BD, Giller EL, Southwick SM. Altered platelet alpha-2-adrenergic receptor affinity states in post-traumatic stress disorder. Am J Psychiatry 144:1511–1512, 1987

Perry BD, Southwick SM, Giller EL: Adrenergic receptor regulation in posttraumatic stress disorder, in Biological Assessment and Treatment of Post Traumatic Stress Disorder. Edited by Giller EL. Washington, DC, American Psychiatric Press, 1990, pp 87–114

Pitman RK: Post-traumatic stress disorder, conditioning, and network theory. Psychiatric Ann 18:182–189, 1988

Pitman RK: Post-traumatic stress disorder, hormones, and memory. Biol Psychiatry 26:221–223, 1989

Pitman RK, Orr SP: Twenty-four hour urinary cortisol and catecholamine excretion in combat-related post-traumatic stress disorder. Biol Psychiatry 27:245–247, 1990

Pitman RK, Orr SP, Forgue DF, et al: Psychophysiologic assessment of posttraumatic stress disorder imagery in Vietnam combat veterans. Arch Gen Psychiatry 44:970–975, 1987

Pitman RK, Orr SP, Forgue DF, et al: Psychophysiologic responses to combat imagery of Vietnam veterans with post-traumatic stress disorder vs. other anxiety disorders. J Abnorm Psychol 99:49–54, 1990a

Pitman RK, van der Kolk BA, Orr SP, et al: Naloxone-reversible analgesic response to combat-related stimuli in post-traumatic stress disorder: a pilot study. Arch Gen Psychiatry 47:541–544, 1990b

Rainey JM, Aleem A, Ortiz A, et al: A laboratory procedure for the induction of flashbacks. Am J Psychiatry 144:1317–1319, 1987

Shestatzky M, Greenberg D, Lerer B. A controlled trial of phenelzine in post traumatic stress disorder. Psychiatry Res 24:149–155, 1988

Smith MA, Davidson J, Ritchie JC, et al: The corticotropin-releasing hormone test in patients with posttraumatic stress disorder. Biol Psychiatry 26:349–355, 1989

van der Kolk BA: The drug treatment of post-traumatic stress disorder. J Affective Disord 13:203–213, 1987

van der Kolk BA, Greenberg MS: The psychobiology of the trauma response: hyperarousal, constriction, and addiction to traumatic reexposure, in Psychological Trauma. Edited by van der Kolk BA. Washington, DC, American Psychiatric Press, 1987, pp 63–87

van der Kolk BA, Greenberg MS, Boyd H, et al. Inescapable shock, neurotransmitters and addiction to trauma: towards a psychobiology of post traumatic stress. Biol Psychiatry 20:314–325, 1985

van der Kolk BA, Pitman RK, Orr SP, et al: Endogenous opioids, stress-induced analgesia, and post-traumatic stress disorder. Psychopharmacol Bull 25:417–422, 1989

van Kammen WB, Christiansen C, van Kammen DP, et al: Sleep and the POW experience: forty years later, in Biological Assessment and Treatment of Post Traumatic Stress Disorder. Edited by Giller EL. Washington, DC, American Psychiatric Press, 1990, pp 159–172

Wolf ME, Alavi A, Mosnaim AD. Posttraumatic stress disorder in Vietnam veterans: clinical and EEG findings; possible therapeutic effects of carbamazephine. Biol Psychiatry 23:642–644, 1988

# Classifications of Posttraumatic Stress Disorder in DSM-IV: Anxiety Disorder, Dissociative Disorder, or Stress Disorder?

**Elizabeth A. Brett, Ph.D.**

***Summary***    The author outlines 4 different options for classifying PTSD. These are 1) retaining it as an anxiety disorder, 2) classifying it as a dissociative disorder, 3) classifying it by etiology as one of a broadly conceived stress category, and 4) classifying it by etiology in a narrowly defined stress category. The various cases are evaluated, with reference to comorbidity, family history, animal models, and other parameters. The author's preference, based on this review, is for recommending a narrowly based etiological classification.

## Statement of the Issue

Posttraumatic stress disorder (PTSD) sits uneasily in its present classification as an anxiety disorder. Evidence for this is, first, the intense controversy in DSM-III-R (American Psychiatric Association 1987) over whether PTSD was an anxiety or dissociative disorder (Brett et al. 1988), and second, the unanimous vote of the DSM-IV Advisory Subcommittee on PTSD to classify PTSD in a new stress response category. In this chapter, I review the empirical evidence for the classification of PTSD as an anxiety disorder and as a dissociative disorder, and evaluate four options for classifying PTSD. These options are: 1) retaining PTSD as an anxiety disorder, 2) classifying PTSD as a dissociative disorder, 3) classifying PTSD in a broadly conceived stress category, Stress Response Disorders, and 4) classifying PTSD in a narrowly defined stress category, Disorders of Extreme Stress Not Elsewhere Classified.

Option 3, the inclusive stress category, is:

### Stress Response Disorder

1. Acute Stress Disorder
2. Posttraumatic Stress Disorder
3. Pathological Grief
4. Uncomplicated Bereavement
5. (Adjustment Disorders as a possibility)

Option 4, the limited stress category, is:

### Disorders of Extreme Stress Not Elsewhere Classified

1. Acute Stress Disorder
2. Posttraumatic Stress Disorder
3. Disorders of Extreme Stress Not Otherwise Specified

# Literature Review

## Method

A comprehensive search of the psychiatric and psychological literature from 1985 to 1989 was conducted using the term *posttraumatic stress disorder.*

With respect to the relationship of PTSD to the dissociative disorders, studies were included only if they investigated subjects with a diagnosis of PTSD or a dissociative disorder. There are a number of studies in the literature reporting reactions to extreme stress in the form of symptoms rather than diagnoses (see Chapter 12), but these studies offer more equivocal evidence for the question of classification.

# PTSD as an Anxiety Disorder

## Results

### Studies of Comorbidity

A series of studies have demonstrated that PTSD frequently co-occurs with one or more additional diagnoses (Davidson et al. 1985, 1991; Escobar et al. 1983; Green et al. 1989; Helzer et al. 1987; Sierles et al. 1983). Table 10–1 shows the design features and sample characteristics of each study; Table 10–2 shows the percentage of PTSD subjects in each study with other diagnoses. The results of the study by Helzer and colleagues are reported as risk ratios for making another diagnosis rather than percentages. As inspection of Table 10–2 demonstrates, PTSD co-occurs most frequently with substance abuse, depression, and anxiety disorders. Although the various studies show one or other of these to be more common, these three categories are the most frequent additional diagnoses.

By examining the predictive ability of war stressors, the study by Green and colleagues (1989) adds a dimension to what in the other studies is a purely descriptive account of co-occurrence. Green and her colleagues found that particular war stressors predict specific combinations of PTSD and other diagnoses. Panic and PTSD was highly predictable by "special assignment tasks," one of several war stressor variables, and the researchers conclude that forms of PTSD characterized by anxiety may have been

Table 10–1.   Design features and sample characteristics of PTSD comorbidity

| Study | Diagnostic Instrument | Type of Sample | Total N | # of PTSD Subjects |
|-------|----------------------|----------------|---------|--------------------|
| Escobar et al. 1983 | DIS | Hispanic outpatients | 41 | 20 |
| Sierles et al. 1983 | SADS, Iowa Structured Patient Interview | Inpatients | 25 | 25 |
| Davidson et al. 1985 | SADS, DSM-III structured interview | Inpatients, outpatients | 36 | 36 |
| Helzer et al. 1987 | DIS | Community | 2,493 | 26 |
| Green et al. 1989 | SADS, DSM-III structured interview | Outpatient community | 200 | 58 |
| Davidson et al. 1991 | DIS | Community | 2,895 | 39 |

Note.   DIS = Diagnostic Interview Schedule (Robins et al. 1981); SADS = Schedule for Affective Disorders and Schizophrenia (Endicott and Spitzer 1978).

Table 10–2.    Percentages of PTSD subjects with comorbid diagnoses in studies of PTSD and comorbidity

| Diagnoses | Escobar et al. 1983 | Sierles et al. 1983 | Davidson et al. 1985 | Helzer et al. 1987 | Green et al. 1989 | Davidson et al. 1991 |
|---|---|---|---|---|---|---|
| Alcohol abuse/dependence | 80 | 64 | 41 | 1.6[*] | 21 | 6.9 |
| Drug abuse/dependence | 50 | 20 | 16 | 2.2[*] | | 9.0 |
| Major depression | 35 | 8 | 41 | 5.7[b*] | 35 | 29.9 |
| Dysthymia | | | | 7.8[*] | | 7.9 |
| Generalized anxiety | | | | | | 53.9 |
| Panic disorder | 5 | | 19[a] | 4.0[*] | 17.6 | 13.6 |
| Social phobia | 50 | | | 3.3[*] | 49.3[c] | 22.3 |
| Simple phobia | 20 | | | | | 50.1 |
| Agoraphobia | 5 | | | | | 31.6 |
| Obsessive-compulsive disorder | 15 | | 3 | 10.1[*] | | 14.5 |
| Somatization disorder | 15 | 8 | | | | 11.7 |

[a] Generalized anxiety, panic and phobic disorder combined.
[b] Major depression, manic depressive disorder and/or mania.
[c] All phobias combined.
[*] Risk ratio.

caused by stressor experiences that themselves involved high levels of anxiety and terror. Interestingly, although major depression occurred often with PTSD, war stressors predicted that particular diagnosis less strongly than other diagnoses. The authors speculate that depression may be a secondary condition developing in response to the chronic stress disorder rather than developing directly in reaction to the stressful event (Green et al. 1989).

### Studies of Family History

Two studies examine familial psychiatric illness in PTSD patients (Davidson et al. 1985, 1989). No clear patterns of illness emerged. In the first study, the only increased morbidity risk for disorder in relatives when comparing PTSD patients ($N = 36$) with depressed and anxious controls is higher alcoholism in siblings of PTSD patients (Davidson et al. 1985). In the second study, the only significant difference in morbidity risk for disorder in relatives comparing the PTSD group ($N = 108$) and depressed, alcoholic, and nonpsychiatric controls is greater depression in the families of depressed probands (Davidson et al. 1989). However, findings in each study suggest some support for a greater genetic link between PTSD and anxiety than between PTSD and depression.

In a study by Davidson and colleagues (1985), the PTSD and generalized anxiety groups have similar proportions of anxiety and depression, whereas the depressed controls show much greater depression and much less anxiety. In their second study, Davidson and colleagues (1989) showed that, when compared with combat-exposed controls, the PTSD group carried greater familial risk of anxiety, whereas the depressed controls showed greater morbidity risk for depression in relatives when compared with the PTSD group. These studies both used information about family members obtained from the proband. Studies using direct interviews of family members are needed.

### Animal Models and Studies of Psychophysiology

In a review of the research on animal models of stress and the physiology of PTSD, Pitman points to two major findings from these investigations: 1) stimuli resembling the traumatic stressor cause sympathetic nervous system hyperresponsivity, and 2) tonic or resting hyperactivity of the sympathetic nervous system characterizes individuals with PTSD and is hypothesized to be a response to the traumatic stressor, although this relationship needs to be more firmly established (see Chapter 9).

## Discussion

At this time, there are no findings demonstrating a strong relationship between PTSD and the anxiety disorders in studies of comorbidity or family history, although arguments have been made that particular findings indicate modest support for some association between anxiety and PTSD. PTSD certainly occurs frequently with diagnoses of substance abuse, depression, and anxiety. Underlying this coexistence of symptoms are complex questions of genetic predisposition, primary and secondary disorders, and the etiologic specificity of stressors.

What are the nosological implications of the work on animal models and psychophysiology? The most important conclusion to be drawn is that it supports the etiological approach to PTSD, as described in DSM-III (American Psychiatric Association 1980) and DSM-III-R (i.e., traumatic stressors cause symptoms of stress). Although these studies indicate some similarity between anxiety disorders and PTSD (e.g., resting sympathetic nervous system hyperreactivity), the similarity is one of pathogenesis (i.e., both disorders may have the same mechanism determining the expression of symptoms). What is different is that in PTSD we can posit an etiological explanation, whereas with the anxiety disorders we must remain with pathogenesis and cannot take the next step to a higher level of explanation. Given that medical disorders can be described on the basis of symptoms, anatomical changes, pathogenesis, and etiology in an ascending order of desirability, the etiological explanation is the preferred one (see Chapter 9).

# PTSD as a Dissociative Disorder

## Results

### *External Validators*

Stutman and Bliss (1985) and Spiegel and colleagues (1988) have both used hypnotizability as a measure of dissociation. Not only was hypnotizability greater in patients with higher levels of PTSD but hypnotizability was greater in PTSD patients than in patients with other disorders (Stutman and Bliss 1985). Of particular note was the finding that hypnotizability was twice as high in patients with PTSD as in patients with generalized anxiety disorder (GAD), suggesting a difference between PTSD and the anxiety disorders on this variable (Spiegel et al. 1988). Overall, both research groups conclude that dissociation increases with greater levels of posttraumatic stress.

Using a more direct measure of dissociative phenomena, the Dissociative Experiences Scale (DES; Bernstein 1986), Marmar and colleagues (C. Marmar et al., unpublished observations, October 1988) found in the clinical subsample of the National Vietnam Veterans Readjustment Study (NVVRS) that dissociation as a trait correlates strongly with a variety of measures of PTSD. In a comparison of patients with complex partial seizures, multiple personality disorder (MPD), and PTSD, Lowenstein and Putnam (1988) found that the MPD and PTSD patients differed significantly from the seizure patients on the DES, and that the MPD and PTSD patients showed similar scores on the scale, with only one of the three subscales showing a significant difference.

In another study using the DES with PTSD, anxious and healthy controls, the investigators found a significant difference between the PTSD and healthy group on dissociation but did not find a significant difference between the PTSD and anxious group on dissociation. On a variety of other measures as well, similarity of scores among the PTSD and anxious groups led the investigators to infer a resemblance in the disorders. A weakness of the study is the small number of subjects ($N = 7$) in the anxious group (Orr et al. 1990).

One study examined the relationship between PTSD and a dissociative event, analgesia: Pitman and colleagues (1990) found that viewing a combat film led to analgesia in PTSD combat veterans but not in non-PTSD combat veterans. The analgesia was naloxone-reversible in the patients with PTSD. This study replicates naloxone reversal of stress-induced analgesia in animals following inescapable shock (Pitman et al. 1990).

### Predictors

In a study of oil rig disaster survivors, Holen (1988) found that dissociation at the moment of the trauma predicted PTSD, psychiatric symptomatology, and adjustment at several follow-up intervals more strongly than objective characteristics of the stressor.

In summary, hypnotizability that is viewed as a dissociative trait was higher in PTSD patients and distinguished patients with GAD from those with PTSD (Spiegel et al. 1988). Dissociation as a trait is found in PTSD and MPD patients (Lowenstein and Putnam 1988) and is higher in PTSD patients than control subjects, although it did not differentiate PTSD and anxious controls (Orr et al. 1990). Dissociation as a trait correlates with a variety of PTSD measures (C. Marmar et al., unpublished observations, October 1988), and dissociation during a traumatic event predicts PTSD and other adjustment measures (Holen 1988). Finally, a physical manifestation of dissociation, analgesia, occurs in PTSD patients in response to a traumatic stimulus and is naloxone-reversible (van der Kolk et al. 1989).

## Discussion

In this section I evaluate the implications of the empirical findings for the relationship of PTSD to the dissociative disorders as well as state and evaluate the argument that intrusion and numbing are dissociative.

What can be concluded from the empirical research? There is not a great deal of systematic research on the relationship of dissociation and PTSD. However, recent research studies indicate that dissociative phenomena may be related to posttraumatic reactions in several ways. Dissociation during a traumatic event or in response to reminders of the event is related to PTSD (Holen 1988; Horowitz 1988), and dissociation as a trait is related to PTSD (Lowenstein and Putnam 1988; C. Marmar et al., unpublished observations, October 1988; Orr et al. 1990; Spiegel et al. 1988; Stutman and Bliss 1985). These studies, which point to a dissociative element in PTSD, are of great interest and are the beginning of what will undoubtedly be a more elaborate and comprehensive empirical examination of differences and similarities between PTSD and the dissociative disorders. At this time, re-classification would require replication of these findings as well as some demonstration that the overlap in symptoms between PTSD and the dissociative disorders is greater or more fundamental than the overlap between PTSD and the anxiety disorders or between PTSD and depressive disorders. Reclassification based on these studies alone does not seem warranted.

Let us look at the argument that PTSD symptoms are dissociative. This position has been taken on the basis of some of the research findings mentioned but has mainly been made on the basis of face validity and inferences about the nature of PTSD and the dissociative disorders. The argument is that a continuum of dissociation exists, with the dissociative disorders at the extreme end. Dissociation is a "disturbance or alteration in the normally integrative functions of identity, memory, or consciousness" (Spiegel et al. 1988, p. 303). The disturbance is said to include an intense focus on certain mental contents with the simultaneous exclusion of others. In addition, "specific memories and associated feelings seem to contain rules excluding other memories and feelings from conscious awareness" (p. 303). Repression differs from dissociation in that the material excluded from awareness does not contain rules about the admissibility of other material to consciousness (Spiegel et al. 1988).

The essential difference, then, between dissociation and other defenses is that dissociation involves rules excluding certain material from awareness. Do the problems with the integration of identities and memories in PTSD contain such rules? Although the notion of sharp divisions of sets of thoughts and affects seem useful when considering the separation of alters in MPD, it is not clear that the lack of integration of memories or identities in PTSD is any different from those in the anxious or depressed person who, when he or she is symptomatic, finds it difficult to gain access to nonanxious or nondepressed states of mind. Thus, although this definition of dissociation is useful when considering extreme behaviors found in the dissociative disorders (and sometimes in PTSD), it is not clear that less severe symptoms such as intrusion and numbing are usefully characterized in this way.

Let us review the pros and cons for PTSD as a dissociative disorder. Arguments for PTSD as a dissociative disorder include:

1. PTSD and the dissociative disorders are reactions to extreme stress, unlike the etiology of the anxiety disorders.
2. PTSD and the dissociative disorders share memory disruptions that are more extreme and of a different quality than those in other anxiety disorders.
3. PTSD and the dissociative disorders share symptoms such as amnesia and dissociative episodes (flashbacks).

Arguments against PTSD as a dissociative disorder include:

1. The anxiety and avoidance in PTSD are symptoms present in the other anxiety disorders.
2. PTSD does not necessarily include amnesia or dissociative episodes. Some of the abrupt and severe forms of dissociation found in the dissociative disorders may and do occur in PTSD, are included in the diagnostic criteria, but are not necessary for the diagnosis.
3. The argument that intrusion and numbing are dissociative is not convincing.

## Options for Classifying PTSD

### Retaining PTSD as an Anxiety Disorder

The arguments for this position are:

1. Psychological symptoms of anxiety and avoidance are shared by PTSD and the anxiety disorders.

2. Certain physiological responses are similar in PTSD and the anxiety disorders.
3. Retaining PTSD as an anxiety disorder is conservative, requiring no change in the nomenclature.

The arguments against this position are:

1. There is not strong empirical evidence suggesting a unique association between PTSD and the anxiety disorders on the basis of comorbidity or family studies.
2. Despite certain similarities in symptoms and psychophysiology, a fundamental difference between PTSD and the anxiety disorders is that PTSD is a disorder defined in terms of its etiology, whereas the etiology of all other anxiety disorders is unknown.
3. The newly proposed Acute Stress Disorder would have to be included in the anxiety disorders if PTSD remained there, creating two stress reaction diagnoses in the midst of the anxiety disorders.

## Classifying PTSD as a Dissociative Disorder

The arguments for classifying PTSD as a dissociative disorder are:

1. PTSD and the dissociative disorders share certain dissociative symptoms such as amnesia and dissociative episodes (flashbacks).
2. The cardinal symptoms of PTSD, intrusion and numbing, are dissociative.
3. The dissociative disorders are believed to be reactions to severe stress, although this has not been as clearly established for the dissociative disorders as for PTSD and is not included in the criteria for the disorders.

The arguments against classifying PTSD as a dissociative disorder are:

1. The justification for considering intrusion and numbing as dissociative phenomena is not convincing.
2. The relationship of the dissociative disorders to extreme stress has not been established as clearly as it has been for PTSD.
3. Although PTSD and the dissociative disorders may be shown to be equally reactions to severe stress, this by itself argues for the creation of

a stress reaction category rather than the inclusion of PTSD in the dissociative disorders.

## Classifying PTSD in a New Category, Stress Response Disorders

Horowitz (M. J. Horowitz, unpublished observations, September 1989) has proposed the following stress reaction category:

### Stress Response Disorders

1. Acute Stress Disorder
2. Posttraumatic Stress Disorder
3. Pathological Grief
4. Uncomplicated Bereavement
5. (Adjustment Disorders as a possibility)

This proposal consists of an initial attempt to describe and differentiate between and among bereavement, pathological grief, and PTSD.

The advantages of this proposal for classifying PTSD are that reactions to stress are classified on an etiologic basis, and one category for stress reactions facilitates differential diagnosis of disorders related to stress. The disadvantages of such a proposal are that the work distinguishing and relating to bereavements, pathological grief, PTSD, and the other potential disorders involving not only different syndromes but stressors of varying severity is not sufficiently advanced to justify reclassification. Also, a comprehensive stress reaction category would have to include groups of disorders such as the dissociative disorders and adjustment disorders that are relatively comfortably classified at this time.

## Classifying PTSD in a New Category, Disorders of Extreme Stress Not Elsewhere Classified

An alternative to the more comprehensive stress category described above in option 3 is:

### Disorders of Extreme Stress Not Elsewhere Classified

1. Acute Stress Disorder
2. Posttraumatic Stress Disorder
3. Disorders of Extreme Stress Not Otherwise Specified

This stress category is restricted to disorders of extreme stress that are not classified elsewhere.

Acute Stress Disorder is a new disorder being proposed for inclusion in DSM-IV. A brief description follows. It is a syndrome occurring in response to the same kind of stressor that precipitates PTSD. The symptoms of the disorder occur during or immediately following (up to several days) the trauma. An episode of the disorder lasts fewer than 4 weeks. As proposed, the disorder contains two diagnostic criteria. Criterion A is the definition of the stressor, which is identical to the definition of the stressor in PTSD. Criterion B is a list of symptoms that include anxiety, hyperarousal, numbing, amnesia, trancelike behavior, derealization, and depersonalization. The symptoms must be severe enough to interfere with social or occupational functioning or with accomplishing tasks such as obtaining assistance and mobilizing resources. There are two important differences between Acute Stress Disorder and PTSD. Acute Stress Disorder is acute and time-limited, and it does not include the reexperiencing symptoms found in PTSD.

Acute Stress Disorder and PTSD, the first two disorders in this new category, are quite similar. The third disorder, Disorder of Extreme Stress Not Otherwise Specified, is included because clinicians and investigators working with diverse populations (including victims of sexual abuse, family violence, torture, and genocidal policies) report stress syndromes similar but not identical to PTSD (see Chapter 12). There is currently no adequate way to diagnose these disorders. Apparently, many clinicians use the PTSD diagnosis for victims of family violence despite the patients' not meeting the diagnostic criteria, because the clinicians believe there is no acceptable alternative.

The advantages of option 4 are as follows:

1. The etiology of the disorders is used as the basis for classification.
2. Stressors of different levels of intensity are not placed in the same category. This category remains one for extreme stressors.
3. For each of the three disorders in this category, the other two will most often be the ones with which the first differential diagnosis will be made.
4. Although this category includes the recognition that other disorders may be precipitated by extreme stress, it allows them to remain classified according to descriptive symptomatology for the time being.
5. The inclusion of an Acute Stress Disorder in addition to PTSD makes

DSM-IV comparable to the more widely used *International Classification of Diseases, 10th Revision* (ICD-10) in this respect.
6. The development of a stress response category recognizes and facilitates work in the field of stress studies.

Disadvantages of the proposal are that classification on the basis of etiology is not in keeping with the descriptive nature of the rest of the nomenclature, and the inclusion of a disorder of extreme stress not otherwise specified will lead to the diagnosis of disorders that are in fact simply cases of mild PTSD.

## Recommendation

It is my opinion that a separate stress response category should be created and that option 4 is preferable to option 3, on the grounds that at this time it is the clearest and most conservative change. However, option 3, the more comprehensive category, is visionary in that it points to issues and questions about disorders and their relation to each other that must be answered within the field (i.e., it indicates the work that awaits us).

## References

American Psychiatric Association: Diagnostic and Statistical Manual of Mental Disorders, 3rd Edition. Washington, DC, American Psychiatric Association, 1980

American Psychiatric Association: Diagnostic and Statistical Manual of Mental Disorders, 3rd Edition, Revised. Washington, DC, American Psychiatric Association, 1987

Bernstein E: Development, reliability and validity of a dissociation scale. J Nerv Ment Dis 174:727–735, 1986

Brett EA, Spitzer RL, Williams JBW: DSM-III-R criteria for posttraumatic stress disorder. Am J Psychiatry 145:1232–1236, 1988

Davidson JRT, Swartz M, Storck M, et al: A diagnostic and family study of posttraumatic stress disorder. Am J Psychiatry 142:90–93, 1985

Davidson JRT, Smith R, Kudler H: Familial psychiatric illness in chronic posttraumatic stress disorder. Compr Psychiatry 30:1–7, 1989

Davidson JRT, Hughes D, Blazer D, et al: Post-traumatic stress disorder in the community: an epidemiological study. Psychol Med 21:1–9, 1991

Endicott J, Spitzer RL: A diagnostic interview: the Schedule for Affective Disorders and Schizophrenia. Arch Gen Psychiatry 35:837–844, 1978

Escobar JI, Randolph ET, Puente G, et al: Post-traumatic stress disorder in Hispanic Vietnam veterans: clinical phenomenology and sociocultural characteristics. J Nerv Ment Dis 171:585–596, 1983

Green BL, Lindy JD, Grace MC, et al: Multiple diagnosis in posttraumatic stress disorder: the role of war stressors. J Nerv Ment Dis 177:329–335, 1989

Helzer JE, Robins LN, McEvoy L: Post-traumatic stress disorder in the general population: findings of the Epidemiologic Catchment Area survey. N Engl J Med 317:1630–1634, 1987

Holen A: Stages of traumatic dreams and psychomotor manifestations. Paper presented at the Fourth Annual Meeting of the Society for Traumatic Stress Studies, Dallas, TX, October 25, 1988

Horowitz MJ: Introduction to Psychodynamics: A New Synthesis. New York, Basic Books, 1988

Lowenstein RJ, Putnam FW: A comparison study of dissociative symptoms in patients with complex partial seizures, MPD, and posttraumatic stress disorder. Dissociation 1:17–23, 1988

Orr SP, Claiborn JM, Altman B, et al: Psychometric profile of PTSD, anxious, and healthy Vietnam veterans: Correlations with psychophysiologic responses. J Consult Clin Psychol 58:329–335, 1990

Pitman RK, van der Kolk BA, Orr SP, et al: Naloxone-reversible analgesic response to combat-related stimuli in post-traumatic stress disorder: a pilot study. Arch Gen Psychiatry 47:541–544, 1990

Robins LN, Helzer JE, Croughan J, et al: National Institute of Mental Health Diagnostic Interview Schedule: its history, characteristics, and validity. Arch Gen Psychiatry 38:381–389, 1981

Sierles FS, Chen J, McFarland RE, et al: Posttraumatic stress disorder and concurrent psychiatric illness: a preliminary report. Am J Psychiatry 140:1177–1179, 1983

Spiegel D, Hunt T, Dondershine HE: Dissociation and hypnotizability in posttraumatic stress disorder. Am J Psychiatry 145:301–305, 1988

Stutman RK, Bliss EL: Posttraumatic stress disorder, hypnotizability, and imagery. Am J Psychiatry 142:741–743, 1985

van der Kolk BA, Greenberg MS, Orr SP, et al: Endogenous opioids, stress induced analgesia, and post traumatic stress disorder. Psychopharmacol Bull 25:417–421, 1989

# Section V:

# Posttraumatic Stress Disorder in Relation to Other Disorders

# ◆ 11 ◆ On The Distinction Between Traumatic Simple Phobia and Posttraumatic Stress Disorder

Richard J. McNally, Ph.D.
Philip A. Saigh, Ph.D.

**Summary** Simple phobia of traumatic origin overlaps with posttraumatic stress disorder (PTSD). The authors describe different ways in which distinction between the two disorders can be blurred. Following a literature review, they conclude that the problem is more definitional than empirical. Options are presented for classifying patients whose symptom picture presents diagnostic difficulty.

## Statement of the Issue

Simple phobias have diverse etiologies. Some develop following harmless but frightening experiences in the to-be phobic situation (e.g., McNally and Steketee 1985); some develop through vicarious learning (e.g., Öst 1987); whereas others develop following traumatic, life-threatening events (e.g., automobile accidents; Munjack 1984). The occurrence of "traumatic simple phobias" raises issues concerning the distinction between these pathological fears and PTSD.

The distinction between simple phobia and PTSD can be blurred in two principal ways. On the one hand, an individual may be exposed to a traumatic stressor meeting Criterion A for PTSD but exhibit only the signs and symptoms of simple phobia. On the other hand, an individual may be exposed to a subtraumatic stressor that does not qualify for Criterion A yet nevertheless exhibit signs and symptoms suggestive of PTSD. For example, Thyer and Curtis (1983) described a woman who accidentally killed a group of frogs while mowing her lawn. Subsequently, she experienced upsetting dreams about the event, insomnia, and fear and avoidance of frog-related stimuli. Although Thyer and Curtis diagnosed her as having simple phobia, Barlow (1988, pp. 497–498) suggested that she might just as easily be diagnosed as having PTSD—had killing frogs satisfied Criterion A.

In this chapter, we discuss issues relevant to the distinction between traumatic simple phobias and PTSD. We review the limited data available and outline diagnostic options for distinguishing between traumatic simple phobia and PTSD.

# Results

Several researchers describe cases of traumatically conditioned phobias. Goorney and O'Connor (1971) assessed the development of "anxiety states" in 97 Royal Air Force aircraft crew members. They noted that 8% developed "symptoms" following the occurrence of an accident involving themselves or a comrade. It is unclear whether DSM-III-R (American Psychiatric Association 1987) simple phobia or PTSD would have been diagnosed in these cases.

Using behavior therapy techniques, Fairbank and colleagues (1981) treated the "posttraumatic startle response" of a 32-year-old woman who survived a head-on automobile accident. Though several people were injured, there were no fatalities. Because the startle response occurred only to discrete highway-related stimuli, it is questionable whether this case constitutes PTSD. Apart from phobic avoidance, no other PTSD symptoms were reported.

Munjack (1984) studied 25 female and 5 male subjects with driving phobias, 20% of whom developed a simple phobia after a collision. Most of the others acquired their phobia after experiencing a panic attack while behind the wheel. There was no mention of PTSD.

In contrast, Kuch and colleagues (1985) diagnosed DSM-III (American Psychiatric Association 1980) PTSD in 22 men and 8 women who sought therapy for driving fears. In each case, their fears emerged after a serious, but nonfatal, accident. Taken together, these findings suggest that collisions are most likely to produce PTSD, whereas other unpleasant experiences (e.g., dizzy spells, panic) are most likely to produce simple phobias without the wide-ranging psychopathology associated with PTSD. Many people, of course, have such experiences without developing any symptoms whatsoever.

Burstein (1984) used imipramine to treat 10 patients whose Impact of Events Scale scores (Horowitz et al. 1979) suggested DSM-III PTSD. Seven of these patients had been in automobile accidents. Details of the cases were not provided. For example, it is unclear whether patients experienced a "mere" conditioning event (e.g., car crash) or whether they witnessed the horrific death of family and friends. The latter would clearly meet DSM-III-R Criterion A, whereas the former need not.

McCaffrey and Fairbank (1985) treated two patients whose DSM-III PTSD stemmed from transportation accidents. The first case involved a 31-year-old man who developed PTSD after being told about a helicopter crash that killed four of his friends. He had previously witnessed such a crash while serving in the military. His PTSD, however, developed only after the second event. The second case involved a 28-year-old woman who (finally) developed PTSD following her fourth automobile accident. The four accidents occurred within a 14-month period.

Gislason and Call (1982) described three children under the age of three who were severely bitten on the face by dogs. These children developed transient fears of dogs and experienced nightmares about being bitten, but none developed PTSD.

Chatoor and colleagues (1988) described five childhood cases of "posttraumatic" choking phobia. Each child became very fearful of choking on food following a gagging incident. Two children also experienced nightmares about choking. Otherwise, PTSD symptoms were absent.

In summary, there are several published cases involving "posttraumatic" simple phobias. Whether simple phobia or PTSD results from exposure to, say, an automobile accident will probably depend on the extent of injury to the victims, preexisting psychopathology in the patient, and other factors in addition to the stressor itself. Kuch (1989), for example, reported that automobile accidents tend to produce more psychopathology in passengers than in drivers, in people who believe they were not responsible for the accident, in people with a history of automobile accidents, and in people with a history of another anxiety disorder.

The distinction between posttraumatic simple phobia and PTSD, however, is more a definitional than an empirical problem. These issues are discussed below.

## Discussion

As noted previously, there are two types of borderline cases that can blur the distinction between simple phobia and PTSD. The first type includes patients who have been exposed to a traumatic stressor but who only exhibit the fear and avoidance symptoms characteristic of simple phobia. The second type includes patients who have been exposed to a subtraumatic stressor but who exhibit the symptoms of PTSD. What are the diagnostic options in these cases?

For the first type, we see no problem with diagnosing simple phobia. In DSM-III-R, simple phobia is diagnosed on a strictly phenomenological basis; etiology is irrelevant. There is no clear evidence that mode of acquisition (i.e., traumatic versus subtraumatic) influences course or response to treatment. Therefore, there is no obvious reason to alter the simple phobia criteria to accommodate etiology.

For the second type, there are four diagnostic options. First, if we suspend the traumatic stressor criterion, then the patient meets criteria for PTSD. Indeed, the DSM-IV PTSD workgroup is considering modifications to the traumatic stressor as a *diagnostic criterion,* is looking at the relation between low magnitude stress and PTSD, and is considering grouping PTSD and related conditions under the rubric of stress-related disorders. On the one hand, this would seem to solve the simple phobia versus PTSD dilemma. On the other hand, it may merely shift the focus of the problem. That is, although problems with Criterion A might be lessened (the problematic etiological criterion would be removed from the PTSD criteria set per se), the entire group of stress-related disorders would be etiologically based, as with the organic mental disorders.

The second option is to classify patients as individuals with simple phobias who display PTSD symptoms without having experienced a traumatic stressor. This option, however, does not do justice to the full range of symptoms. The fear-related symptoms would be captured by a simple phobia diagnosis, but the emotional numbing and reexperiencing symptoms would not.

The third option is to classify these patients as cases of adjustment disorder. Indeed, strict interpretation of DSM-III-R indicates the appropriateness of this diagnosis rather than a diagnosis of PTSD or simple phobia. Unfortunately, the adjustment disorder diagnosis is not very illuminating concerning the specific symptoms exhibited by such patients.

The fourth option is to classify these patients as cases of anxiety disorder not otherwise specified. Because this is a residual category, it is the least satisfying solution.

## Conclusions

Concerns about the distinction between simple phobia and PTSD arise because the former is diagnosed on descriptive criteria, whereas the latter is diagnosed on both descriptive and etiological criteria. Thus, a patient who meets the descriptive criteria for PTSD but who fails to meet the etiological criterion (e.g., traumatic stressor) cannot be classified as a PTSD case. Consequently, the distinction between simple phobia and PTSD is primarily definitional rather than empirical. If Criterion A remains unchanged in the PTSD criteria set, then individuals whose "PTSD" symptoms emerge after exposure to nontraumatic stressors should receive an adjustment disorder diagnosis rather than a simple phobia or a PTSD diagnosis under current DSM-III-R rules. Individuals who develop only phobic symptoms following exposure to a traumatic stressor lying outside the range of usual human experience should receive a diagnosis of simple phobia.

## References

American Psychiatric Association: Diagnostic and Statistical Manual of Mental Disorders, 3rd Edition. Washington, DC, American Psychiatric Association, 1980

American Psychiatric Association: Diagnostic and Statistical Manual of Mental Disorders, 3rd Edition, Revised. Washington, DC, American Psychiatric Association, 1987

Barlow DH: Anxiety and Its Disorders. New York, Guilford, 1988

Burstein A: Treatment of post-traumatic stress disorder with imipramine. Psychosomatics 25:681–687, 1984

Chatoor I, Conley C, Dickson L: Food refusal after an incident of choking: a post-traumatic eating disorder. J Am Acad Child Adolesc Psychiatry 27:105–110, 1988

Fairbank JA, DeGood DE, Jenkins CW. Behavioral treatment of a persistent post-traumatic startle response. J Behav Ther Exp Psychiatry 12:321–324, 1981

Gislason IL, Call JD: Dog bite in infancy: trauma and personality development. J Am Acad Child Psychiatry 21:203–207, 1982

Goorney B, O'Connor PJ: Anxiety associated with flying: a retrospective survey of military aircrew psychiatric casualties. Br J Psychiatry 119:156–166, 1971

Horowitz M, Wilner N, Alvarez W: Impact of Events Scale: a measure of subjective stress. Psychosom Med 41:209–218, 1979

Kuch K: Enigmatic disability after minor accidents. Modern Medicine of Canada 44:38–41, 1989

Kuch K, Swinson RP, Kirby M. Post-traumatic stress disorder after car accidents. Can J Psychiatry 30:426–427, 1985

McCaffrey RJ, Fairbank JA: Behavioral assessment and treatment of accident-related posttraumatic stress disorder: two case studies. Behavior Therapy 16:406–416, 1985

McNally RJ, Steketee GS: The etiology and maintenance of severe animal phobias. Behav Res Ther 23:431–435, 1985

Munjack DJ: The onset of driving phobias. J Behav Ther Exp Psychiatry 15:305–308, 1984

Öst LG: Age of onset in different phobias. J Abnorm Psychol 96:223–229, 1987

Thyer BA, Curtis GC: The repeated pretest-posttest single-subject experiment: a new design for empirical clinical practice. J Behav Ther Exp Psychiatry 14:311–315, 1983

# ◆ 12 ◆ Sequelae of Prolonged and Repeated Trauma: Evidence for a Complex Posttraumatic Syndrome (DESNOS)

Judith L. Herman, M.D.

**Summary**     The author reviews the evidence to support a more complex type of posttraumatic stress reaction, occurring characteristically in victims of prolonged, repeated interpersonal violence or victimization. This syndrome is provisionally called Disorder of Extreme Stress Not Otherwise Specified (DESNOS). Three dimensions are described: 1) symptomatology, 2) character traits, and 3) vulnerability to repeated harm. Multiple symptoms, excessive somatization, dissociation, and changes of affect are described. Pathological relationship and identity formations are noted to occur. The occurrence of repeated harm-seeking behavior is also noted and discussed. Recommendations are given for further testing of this proposed disorder.

## Statement of the Issue

The current diagnostic formulation of PTSD derives primarily from observations of survivors of relatively circumscribed traumatic events: combat, disaster, and rape. It has been suggested that this formulation fails to capture the protean symptomatic manifestations of prolonged, repeated

Adapted from *Trauma and Recovery* by Judith L. Herman, M.D., published by Basic Books in April 1992.

trauma, or the extensive alterations of personality that occur during protracted captivity. This chapter reviews evidence for the existence of a more complex form of posttraumatic disorder in survivors of prolonged, repeated trauma. A preliminary formulation of this complex posttraumatic syndrome is currently under consideration for inclusion in DSM-IV under the name of DESNOS (Disorders of Extreme Stress Not Otherwise Specified).

# Methodology

Because the proposed diagnostic entity has not been previously named, the usual methodology of a systematic literature search could not be employed. In the course of a larger work in progress, literature on survivors of prolonged political, domestic, or sexual victimization has been scanned (Herman 1992). The literature reviewed included first-person accounts of survivors themselves, descriptive clinical literature, and (where available) more rigorously designed clinical studies. Particular attention was focused on those observations of the sequelae of prolonged victimization that did not fit readily into the existing criteria for PTSD.

# Results

## Clinical Recognition of a DESNOS-Like Entity

The concept of a spectrum of posttraumatic disorders has been suggested independently by many major contributors to the field. Kolb (1989) writes of the "heterogeneity" of PTSD, observing that "PTSD is to psychiatry as syphilis was to medicine. At one time or another PTSD may appear to mimic every personality disorder," and notes further that "it is those threatened over long periods of time who suffer the long-standing severe personality disorganization" (pp. 811–812). Krystal (1968a) quotes Niederland (1968) who, on the basis of his work with survivors of the Nazi Holocaust, observes that "the concept of traumatic neurosis does not appear sufficient to cover the multitude and severity of clinical manifestations" of the survivor syndrome (p. 314). Krystal also quotes Tanay who, working with the same population, notes that "the psychopathology may be hidden in characterological changes that are manifest only in disturbed object relationships and attitudes towards work, the world, man and God" (Krystal 1968a, p. 221). Similarly, Kroll and colleagues (1989), on the basis of work with Southeast Asian refugees, suggest the need for an "expanded concept of PTSD that takes into account the observations [of the effects of] severe, prolonged, and/or massive psychological and physical traumata" (p. 1596). Horowitz (1986) also suggests the concept of a "posttraumatic character disorder" (p. 49).

Clinicians working with survivors of childhood abuse also invoke the need for an expanded diagnostic concept. Gelinas (1983) describes the disguised presentation of the survivor of childhood sexual abuse as a patient with chronic depression complicated by dissociative symptoms, substance abuse, impulsivity, self-mutilation, and suicidality. She formulates the underlying psychopathology as a complicated traumatic neurosis. Goodwin (1988) conceptualizes the sequelae of prolonged childhood abuse as a severe posttraumatic syndrome that includes fugue and other dissociative states, ego fragmentation, affective and anxiety disorders, reenactment and revictimization, somatization, and suicidality.

Clinical observations identify three broad areas of disturbance that transcend simple PTSD. The first is symptomatic: the symptom picture in survivors of prolonged trauma often appears to be more complex, diffuse, and tenacious than in simple PTSD. The second is characterological: survivors of prolonged abuse develop characteristic personality changes, including deformations of relatedness and identity. The third area involves the survivor's vulnerability to repeated harm, both self-inflicted and at the hands of others.

## Symptomatic Sequelae of Prolonged Victimization

### Multiplicity of Symptoms

The pathological environment of prolonged abuse fosters the development of a prodigious array of psychiatric symptoms. A history of abuse, particularly in childhood, appears to be one of the major factors predisposing a person to become a psychiatric patient. Although only a minority of survivors of chronic childhood abuse become psychiatric patients, a large proportion (40–70%) of adult psychiatric patients are survivors of abuse (Briere and Runtz 1987; Briere and Zaidi 1989; Bryer et al. 1987; Carmen et al. 1984; Jacobson and Richardson 1987).

Survivors who become patients present with a multitude of complaints. Their general levels of distress are higher than those of patients who do not have histories of abuse. Detailed inventories of their symptoms reveal significant pathology in multiple domains: somatic, cognitive, affective, behavioral, and relational. Bryer and his colleagues (1987), studying psychiatric inpatients, report that women with histories of physical or sexual abuse have significantly higher scores than other patients on standardized measures of somatization, depression, general and phobic anxiety, interpersonal sensitivity, paranoia, and "psychoticism" (dissociative symptoms were not measured specifically). Briere (1988), studying outpatients at a crisis intervention service, reports that survivors of childhood abuse display significantly more insomnia, sexual dysfunction, dissociation, anger, suicidality, self-mutilation, drug addiction, and alcoholism than other patients. Perhaps the most impressive finding of studies employing a "symptom checklist" approach is the sheer length of the list of symptoms found to be significantly related to a history of childhood abuse (Browne and Finkelhor 1986). From this wide array of symptoms, three categories have been selected that do not readily fall within the classic diagnostic criteria for PTSD: the somatic, dissociative, and affective sequelae of prolonged trauma.

### Somatization

Repetitive trauma appears to amplify and generalize the physiologic symptoms of PTSD. Chronically traumatized people are hypervigilant, anxious, and agitated, without any recognizable baseline state of calm or comfort (Hilberman 1980). Over time, they begin to complain, not only of insomnia, startle reactions, and agitation, but also of numerous other somatic symptoms. Tension headaches, gastrointestinal disturbances, and abdominal, back, or pelvic pain are extremely common. Survivors also frequently complain of tremors, choking sensations, or nausea. In clinical studies of survivors of the Nazi Holocaust, psychosomatic reactions were found to be practically universal (DeLoos 1990; Hoppe 1968; Krystal 1968b). Similar observations are now reported in refugees from concentration camps in Southeast Asia (Kinzie et al. 1990; Kroll et al. 1989). Some survivors may conceptualize the damage of their prolonged captivity primarily in somatic terms. Nonspecific somatic symptoms appear to be extremely durable and may in fact increase over time (van der Ploerd 1989).

The clinical literature also suggests an association between somatization disorders and childhood trauma. Briquet's initial descriptions of the disorder that now bears his name are filled with anecdotal references to domestic violence and child abuse. In a study of 87 children under age 12 with hysteria, Briquet (1859) noted that one-third had been "habitually mistreated or held constantly in fear or had been directed harshly by their parents" (p. 112). In another 10%, he attributed the children's symptoms to traumatic experiences other than parental abuse (Mai and Merskey 1980). A recent controlled study of 60 women with somatization disorder found that 55% had been sexually molested in childhood, usually by relatives. The study focused only on early sexual experiences; patients were not asked about physical abuse or about the more general climate of violence in their families (Morrison 1989). Systematic investigation of the childhood histories of patients with somatization disorder has yet to be undertaken.

### Dissociation

People in captivity become adept practitioners of the arts of altered consciousness. Through the practice of dissociation, voluntary thought suppression, minimization, and sometimes outright denial, they learn to alter an unbearable reality. Prisoners frequently instruct one another in the induction of trance states. These methods are consciously applied to withstand hunger, cold, and pain (Partnoy 1986; Scharansky 1988). During prolonged confinement and isolation, some prisoners are able to develop trance capabilities ordinarily seen only in extremely hypnotizable people, including the ability to form positive and negative hallucinations and the ability to dissociate parts of the personality (Russell 1989; Wechsler 1989). Disturbances in time sense, memory, and concentration are almost universally reported (Allodi 1985; Kinzie et al. 1984; Tennant et al. 1986). Alterations in time sense begin with the obliteration of the future but eventually progress to the obliteration of the past (Levi 1961). The rupture in continuity between present and past frequently persists even after the prisoner is released. The prisoner may give the appearance of returning to ordinary time while psychologically remaining bound in the timelessness of the prison (Jaffe 1968).

In survivors of prolonged childhood abuse, these dissociative capacities are developed to the extreme. Shengold (1989) describes the "mind-fragmenting operations" elaborated by abused children in order to preserve

"the delusion of good parents" (p. 26). He notes the "establishment of isolated divisions of the mind in which contradictory images of the self and of
the parents are never permitted to coalesce" (p. 26). The virtuoso feats of
dissociation seen, for example, in multiple personality disorder (MPD), are
almost always associated with a childhood history of massive and prolonged
abuse (Putnam 1989; Putnam et al. 1986 Ross et al. 1990). A similar association between severity of childhood abuse and extent of dissociative symptomatology has been documented in subjects with borderline personality
disorder (BPD; Herman et al. 1989).

### Affective Changes

There are people with very strong and secure belief systems who can en-
dure the ordeals of prolonged abuse and emerge with their faith intact.
But these are the extraordinary few. The majority experience the bitter-
ness of being forsaken by man and God (Wiesel 1960). These staggering
psychological losses most commonly result in a tenacious state of depression. Protracted depression is reported as the most common finding in
virtually all clinical studies of chronically traumatized people (Hilberman
1980; Kinzie et al. 1984; Krystal 1968a; Tennant et al. 1986; Walker 1979).
Every aspect of the experience of prolonged trauma combines to aggra-
vate depressive symptoms. The chronic hyperarousal and intrusive symptoms of PTSD fuse with the vegetative symptoms of depression,
producing what Niederland (1968) calls the survivor triad of insomnia,
nightmares, and psychosomatic complaints. The dissociative symptoms
of PTSD merge with the concentration difficulties of depression. The paralysis of initiative of chronic trauma combines with the apathy and helplessness of depression. The disruptions in attachments of chronic trauma
reinforce the isolation and withdrawal of depression. The debased self-
image of chronic trauma fuels the guilty ruminations of depression, and
the loss of faith suffered in chronic trauma merges with the hopelessness
of depression.

The intense anger of the imprisoned person also adds to the depressive
burden (Hilberman 1980). During captivity, prisoners cannot express their
humiliated rage at the perpetrator; to do so would jeopardize their survival.
Even after release, prisoners continue to fear retribution and are slow to
express their rage against their captors. Moreover, they are left with a burden
of unexpressed rage against all those who remained indifferent to their fate

and who failed to help them. Efforts to control this rage may further exacerbate the victim's social withdrawal and paralysis of initiative. Occasional outbursts of rage against others may further alienate the victim and prevent the restoration of relationships, and internalization of rage may result in a malignant self-hatred and chronic suicidality. Epidemiologic studies of returned prisoners of war (POWs) consistently document increased mortality as the result of homicide, suicide, and suspicious accidents (Segal et al. 1976). Studies of battered women similarly report a tenacious suicidality. In one clinical series of 100 battered women, 42% had attempted suicide (Gayford 1975).

Although major depression is frequently diagnosed in survivors of prolonged abuse, the connection with trauma is frequently lost. Patients are incompletely treated when the traumatic origins of the intractable depression are not recognized (Kinzie et al. 1990).

## Characterological Sequelae of Prolonged Victimization

### Pathological Changes in Relationship

Chronic, repetitive trauma can occur only where the victim is in a state of captivity, unable to flee, and under the control of the perpetrator. Examples of such conditions include prisons, concentration camps, and slave labor camps. Such conditions also exist in some religious cults, in brothels and other institutions of organized sexual exploitation, and in some families. In situations of captivity, the perpetrator becomes the most powerful person in the life of the victim, and the psychology of the victim is shaped by the actions and beliefs of the perpetrator.

The methods that enable one human being to control another are remarkably consistent. The accounts of battered women, abused children, hostages, political prisoners, and survivors of concentration camps from every corner of the globe have an uncanny sameness. Drawing upon the testimony of political prisoners from widely differing cultures, Amnesty International published a "chart of coercion," describing these methods in detail (Amnesty International 1973; Biederman 1957; Farber et al. 1957). The methods of establishing control over another person are based on the systematic, repetitive infliction of psychological trauma. These methods are designed to instill terror and helplessness, to destroy the victim's sense of self in relation to others, and to foster a pathologic attachment to the perpetrator.

Although violence is a universal method of instilling terror, the threat of death or serious harm, either to the victim or to others close to him or her, is much more frequent than actual violence. Fear is also increased by unpredictable outbursts of violence and by inconsistent enforcement of trivial demands and petty rules. In addition to inducing terror, the perpetrator seeks to destroy the victim's sense of autonomy. This is achieved by control of the victim's body and bodily functions. Deprivation of food, sleep, shelter, exercise, personal hygiene, or privacy are common practices. Once the perpetrator has established this degree of control, he or she becomes a potential source of solace as well as humiliation. The capricious granting of small indulgences may undermine the psychological resistance of the victim far more effectively than unremitting deprivation and fear.

As long as the victim maintains strong relationships with others, the perpetrator's power is limited; invariably, therefore, the perpetrator seeks to isolate the victim. The perpetrator will not only attempt to prohibit communication and material support but will also try to destroy the victim's emotional ties to others. The final step in the "breaking" of the victim is not completed until he or she has been forced to betray the most basic attachments, by witnessing or participating in crimes against others.

As the victim is isolated, he or she becomes increasingly dependent upon the perpetrator, not only for survival and basic bodily needs but also for information and even for emotional sustenance. Prolonged confinement in fear of death and in isolation reliably produces a bond of identification between captor and victim (Strentz 1982; Symonds, 1982). This is the "traumatic bonding" that occurs in hostages who come to view their captors as their saviors and to fear and hate their rescuers. Symonds (1982, p. 99) describes this process as an enforced regression to "psychological infantilism" that "compels victims to cling to the very person who is endangering their life." The same traumatic bonding may occur between a battered woman and her abuser (Dutton and Painter 1981; Graham et al. 1988) or between an abused child and abusive parent (Herman 1981). Similar experiences are also reported by people who have been inducted into totalitarian religious cults (Halperin 1983; Lifton 1987).

With increased dependency on the perpetrator comes a constriction in initiative and planning. Prisoners who have not been entirely "broken" do not give up the capacity for active engagement with their environment. On the contrary, they often approach the small daily tasks of survival with extraordinary ingenuity and determination. But the field of initiative is increasingly narrowed within confines dictated by the perpetrator. The prisoner no longer thinks of how to escape, but rather of how to stay alive or how to make captivity more bearable. This narrowing in the range of initiative becomes habitual with prolonged captivity and must be unlearned after the prisoner is liberated (testimony of Rosencof in Weschler 1989).

Because of this constriction in the capacities for active engagement with the world, chronically traumatized people are often described as passive or helpless. Some theorists have in fact applied the concept of "learned helplessness" to the situation of battered women and other chronically traumatized people (Flannery 1987; Walker 1979). Prolonged captivity undermines or destroys the ordinary sense of a relatively safe sphere of initiative, in which there is some tolerance for trial and error. To the chronically traumatized person, any independent action is insubordination, which carries the risk of dire punishment.

The sense that the perpetrator is still present, even after liberation, signifies a major alteration in the victim's relational world. The enforced relationship, which of necessity monopolizes the victim's attention during captivity, becomes part of the victim's inner life and continues to engross him or her after release. In political prisoners, this continued relationship may take the form of a brooding preoccupation with the criminal careers of specific perpetrators or with more abstract concerns about the unchecked forces of evil in the world. Released prisoners continue to track their captors and to fear them (Krystal 1968a). In sexual, domestic, and religious cult prisoners, this continued relationship may take a more ambivalent form: the victim may continue to fear the former captor and to expect that this person will eventually hunt him or her down; the victim may also feel empty, confused, and worthless without the captor (Walker 1979).

Even after the victim has escaped, it is not possible simply to reconstitute relationships of the sort that existed prior to captivity. All relationships are now viewed through the lens of extremity. Just as there is no range of moderate engagement or risk for initiative, there is no range of moderate engagement or risk for relationship. The survivor approaches all relationships as though questions of life and death are at stake, oscillating between intense attachment and terrified withdrawal.

In survivors of childhood abuse, these disturbances in relationship are further amplified. Oscillations in attachment, with formation of intense, unstable relationships, are frequently observed. These disturbances are described most fully in patients with BPD, the majority of whom have extensive histories of childhood abuse. A recent empirical study, confirming a vast literature of clinical observations, outlines in detail the specific pattern of relational difficulties. Borderline patients find it very hard to tolerate being alone but are also exceedingly wary of others. Terrified of abandonment on the one hand and of domination on the other, they oscillate between extremes of abject submissiveness and furious rebellion (Melges and Swartz 1989). They tend to form "special" dependent relations with idealized caretakers in which ordinary boundaries are not observed (Zanarini et al. 1990). Very similar patterns are described in patients with MPD, including the tendency to develop intense, highly "special" relationships ridden with boundary violations, conflict, and potential for exploitation (Kluft 1990).

### Pathological Changes in Identity

Subjection to a relationship of coercive control produces profound alterations in the victim's identity. All the structures of the self—the image of the body, the internalized images of others, and the values and ideals that lend a sense of coherence and purpose—are invaded and systematically broken down. In many totalitarian systems, this process reaches the extent of taking away the victim's name. Although victims of a single acute trauma may say they are "not themselves" since the event, victims of chronic trauma may lose the sense that they have a self. Survivors may describe themselves as reduced to a nonhuman life form (Lovelace and McGrady 1980; Timerman 1988). Niederland, in his clinical observations of concentration camp survivors, noted that alterations of personal identity were a constant feature of the survivor syndrome. Although the majority of his patients complained, "I am now a different person," the most severely harmed stated simply, "I am not a person" (Niederland 1968).

Survivors of childhood abuse develop even more complex deformations of identity. A malignant sense of the self as contaminated, guilty, and evil is widely observed. Fragmentation in the sense of self is also common, reaching its most dramatic extreme in MPD. Ferenczi, writing in 1933, described the atomization of the abused child's personality (Ferenczi 1955). Rieker and Carmen (1986) describe the central pathology in victimized children as a disordered and fragmented identity deriving from accommodations to the judgments of others. Disturbances in identity formation are also characteristic of patients with borderline disorders and MPD, the majority of whom have childhood histories of severe trauma. In MPD, the fragmentation of the self into dissociated alters is, of course, the central feature of the disorder (Bliss 1986; Putnam 1989). Patients with BPD, though they lack the dissociative capacity to form fragmented alters, have similar difficulties in the formation of an integrated identity. An unstable sense of self is recognized as one of the major diagnostic criteria for BPD, and the "splitting" of inner representations of self and others is considered by some theorists to be the central underlying pathology of the disorder (Kernberg 1967).

### Repetition of Harm Following Prolonged Victimization

Repetitive phenomena have been widely noted to be sequelae of severe trauma. The topic has been recently reviewed in depth by van der Kolk (1989). The phenomenon of repeated victimization appears to be specifically associated with histories of prolonged childhood abuse. Wide-scale epidemiologic studies provide strong evidence that survivors of childhood abuse are at increased risk for repeated abuse in adult life. For example, the risk of rape, sexual harassment, and battering, though very high for all women, is approximately doubled for survivors of childhood sexual abuse (Russell 1986).

In the most extreme cases, survivors of childhood abuse may find themselves reenacting the abuse, either in the role of perpetrator or passive bystander. Burgess and colleagues (1984), for example, report that children who had been exploited in a sex ring for more than 1 year were likely to adopt the belief system of the perpetrators and to become exploitative toward others. A history of prolonged childhood abuse does appear to be a risk factor for becoming an abuser (especially in men; Herman 1988) and for marriage to an abusive mate (especially in women; Goodwin et al. 1982). It should be noted, however, that contrary to the popular notion of a "generational cycle of abuse," the great majority of survivors do not abuse others (Kaufman and Zigler 1987). For the sake of their children, survivors frequently mobilize caring and protective capacities that they have never been able to extend to themselves (Coons 1985).

Deliberate self-injury also seems to be strongly associated with a history of childhood abuse. Self-mutilation, which is rarely seen after a single acute trauma, is a common sequel of protracted childhood abuse (Briere 1988). Our own data indicate that self-injury and other paroxysmal forms of attack on the body develop most commonly in those victims whose abuse began early in childhood (Herman et al. 1990).

These repetitive phenomena call for great care in interpretation. For too long, the clinical literature has simply reflected the crude social judgment that survivors "ask for" and derive gratification from abuse. Earlier concepts of masochism or repetition compulsion might be more usefully supplanted by the concept of a complex traumatic syndrome.

## Recommendations

The review of the literature offers extensive but unsystematized empirical support for the concept of a complex posttraumatic syndrome (DESNOS) in survivors of prolonged, repeated victimization. This syndrome appears to be sufficiently distinct from simple PTSD to warrant systematic field trials.

The current conceptualization of DESNOS was developed primarily by clinicians working with survivors of domestic and sexual abuse. Input should be sought from those working primarily with survivors of political persecution and imprisonment before a more final picture is completed.

If the data from field trials validate the concept of DESNOS, this would further support the recommendation, set forth by Brett (see Chapter 10), for the classification of a spectrum of posttraumatic disorders within a separate category in DSM-IV. This proposed spectrum would include Acute Stress Disorder, PTSD, and DESNOS.

## References

Allodi F: Physical and psychiatric effects of torture: two medical studies, in The Breaking of Bodies and Minds: Torture, Psychiatric Abuse, and the Health Professions. Edited by Stover E, Nightingale EO. New York, Freeman, 1985, pp 58–78

Amnesty International: Report on Torture. New York, Farrar, Straus & Giroux, 1973

Biederman AD: Communist attempts to elicit false confessions from Air Force prisoners of war. Bull N Y Acad Med 33:616–625, 1957

Bliss EL: Multiple Personality, Allied Disorders, and Hypnosis. New York, Oxford University Press, 1986

Briere J: Long-term clinical correlates of childhood sexual victimization. Ann N Y Acad Sciences 528:327–334, 1988

Briere J, Runtz M: Post sexual abuse trauma: data and implications for clinical practice. Journal of Interpersonal Violence 2:367–379, 1987

Briere J, Zaidi LY: Sexual abuse histories and sequelae in female psychiatric emergency room patients. Am J Psychiatry 146:1602–1606, 1989

Briquet P: Traité de L'Hysterie. Paris, J B Bailliere et Fils, 1859

Browne A, Finkelhor D: Impact of child sexual abuse: a review of the literature. Psychol Bull 99:66–77, 1986

Bryer JB, Nelson BA, Miller JB, et al: Childhood sexual and physical abuse as factors in adult psychiatric illness. Am J Psychiatry 144:1426–1430, 1987

Burgess AW, Hartman CE, McCausland MP, et al: Response patterns in children and adolescents exploited through sex rings and pornography. Am J Psychiatry 141:656–662, 1984

Carmen EH, Rieker PP, Mills T: Victims of violence and psychiatric illness. Am J Psychiatry 141:378–383, 1984

Coons PM: Children of parents with multiple personality disorder, in Childhood Antecedents of Multiple Personality Disorder. Edited by Kluft RP. Washington, DC, American Psychiatric Press, 1985, pp 151–166

DeLoos W: Psychosomatic manifestations of chronic PTSD, in Posttraumatic Stress Disorder: Etiology, Phenomenology, and Treatment. Edited by Wolf ME, Mosnaim AD. Washington, DC, American Psychiatric Press, 1990, pp 94–105

Dutton D, Painter SL: Traumatic bonding: the development of emotional attachments in battered women and other relationships of intermittent abuse. Victimology 6:139–155, 1981

Farber IE, Harlow HF, West LJ: Brainwashing, conditioning, and DDD (debility, dependency, and dread). Sociometry 23:120–147, 1957

Ferenczi S: Confusion of tongues between adults and the child: the language of tenderness and of passion, in Final Contributions to the Problems and Methods of Psychoanalysis. Edited by Ferenczi S. New York, Basic Books, 1955, pp 155–167

Flannery R: From victim to survivor: a stress management approach in the treatment of learned helplessness, in Psychological Trauma. Edited by van der Kolk BA. Washington, DC, American Psychiatric Press, 1987, pp 217–232

Gayford JJ: Wife-battering: a preliminary survey of 100 cases. BMJ 1:194–197, 1975

Gelinas D: The persistent negative effects of incest. Psychiatry 46:312–332, 1983

Goodwin J: Evaluation and treatment of incest victims and their families: a problem oriented approach, in Modern Perspectives in Psycho-Social Pathology. Edited by Howells JG. New York, Brunner/Mazel, 1988

Goodwin J, McMarty T, DiVasto P: Physical and sexual abuse of the children of adult incest victims, in Sexual Abuse: Incest Victims and their Families. Edited by Goodwin J. Boston, MA, John Wright, 1982, pp 139–154

Graham DL, Rawlings E, Rimini N: Survivors of terror: battered women, hostages, and the Stockholm syndrome, in Feminist Perspectives on Wife Abuse. Edited by Yllo K, Bograd M. Beverly Hills, CA, Sage, 1988, pp 217–233

Halperin DA: Group processes in cult affiliation and recruitment, in Psychodynamic Perspectives on Religion, Sect, and Cult. Edited by Halperin DA. Boston, MA, John Wright, 1983

Herman JL: Father-Daughter Incest. Cambridge, MA, Harvard University Press, 1981

Herman JL: Considering sex offenders: a model of addiction. Signs: Journal of Women in Culture and Society 13:695–724, 1988

Herman JL: Trauma and Recovery. New York, Basic Books, 1992

Herman JL, Perry JC, van der Kolk BA: Childhood trauma in borderline personality disorder. Am J Psychiatry 146:490–495, 1989

Herman JL, Perry JC, van der Kolk BA: Trauma and neglect in borderline personality disorder. Paper presented at the Annual Meeting of the American Psychiatric Association, New York, May 1990

Hilberman E: The "wife-beater's wife" reconsidered. Am J Psychiatry 137:1336–1347, 1980

Hoppe KD: Resomatization of affects in survivors of persecution. Int J Psychoanal 49:324–326, 1968

Horowitz MJ, Wilner N: Field studies on the impact of life events, in Stress Response Syndromes. Edited by Horowitz MJ. Northvale, NJ, Jason Aronson, 1986, pp 43–68

Jacobson A, Richardson B: Assault experiences of 100 psychiatric inpatients: evidence of the need for routine inquiry. Am J Psychiatry 144:908–913, 1987

Jaffe R: Dissociative phenomena in former concentration camp inmates. Int J Psychoanal 49:310–312, 1968

Kaufman J, Zigler E: Do abused children become abusive parents? Am J Orthopsychiatry 57:186–192, 1987

Kernberg O: Borderline personality organization. J Am Psychoanal Assoc 15:641–685, 1967

Kinzie JD, Fredrickson RH, Ben R, et al: PTSD among survivors of Cambodian concentration camps. Am J Psychiatry 141:645–650, 1984

Kinzie JD, Boehnlein NK, Leung PK, et al: The prevalence of posttraumatic stress disorder and its clinical significance among Southeast Asian refugees. Am J Psychiatry 147:913–917, 1990

Kluft RP: Incest and subsequent revictimization: the case of therapist-patient sexual exploitation, with a description of the sitting duck syndrome, in Incest-Related Syndromes of Adult Psychopathology. Edited by Kluft RP. Washington, DC, American Psychiatric Press, 1990, pp 263–288

Kolb LC: Letter to the editor. Am J Psychiatry 146:811–812, 1989

Kroll J, Habenicht M, Mackenzie T, et al: Depression and posttraumatic stress disorder in Southeast Asian refugees. Am J Psychiatry 146:1592–1597, 1989

Krystal H (ed): Massive Psychic Trauma. New York, International Universities Press, 1968a, p 314

Krystal H: Clinical observations of the survivor syndrome, in Massive Psychic Trauma. Edited by Krystal H. New York, International Universities Press, 1968b, pp 327–348

Levi P: Survival in Auschwitz: the Nazi Assault on Humanity (1958). Translated by Woolf S. New York, Collier, 1961

Lifton RJ: Cults: religious totalism and civil liberties, in The Future of Immortality and Other Essays for a Nuclear Age. Edited by Lifton RJ. New York, Basic Books, 1987

Lovelace L, McGrady M: Ordeal. Secaucus, NJ, Citadel, 1980

Mai FM, Merskey H: Briquet's treatise on hysteria: synopsis and commentary. Arch Gen Psychiatry 37:1401–1405, 1980

Melges FT, Swartz MS: Oscillations of attachment in borderline personality disorder. Am J Psychiatry 146:1115–1120, 1989

Morrison J: Childhood sexual histories of women with somatization disorder. Am J Psychiatry 146:239–241, 1989

Niederland WF: Clinical observations on the "survivor syndrome." Int J Psychoanal 49:313–315, 1968

Partnoy A: The Little School: Tales of Disappearance and Survival in Argentina. San Francisco, CA, Cleis Press, 1986

Putnam FW: Diagnosis and Treatment of Multiple Personality Disorder. New York, Guilford, 1989

Putnam FW, Guroff JJ, Silberman EK, et al: The clinical phenomenology of multiple personality disorder: review of 100 recent cases. J Clin Psychiatry 47:285–293, 1986

Rieker PP, Carmen E (Hilberman): The victim-to-patient process: the disconfirmation and transformation of abuse. Am J Orthopsychiatry 56:360–370, 1986

Ross CA, Miller SD, Reagor R, et al: Structured interview data on 102 cases of multiple personality disorder from four centers. Am J Psychiatry 147:596–601, 1990

Russell DEH: The Secret Trauma. New York, Basic Books, 1986

Russell DEH: Lives of Courage: Women for a New South Africa. New York, Basic Books, 1989

Scharansky N: Fear No Evil. Translated by Hoffman S. New York, Random House, 1988

Segal J, Hunter EJ, Segal Z: Universal consequences of captivity: stress reactions among divergent populations of prisoners of war and their families. International Journal of Social Science 28:593–609, 1976

Shengold L: Soul Murder: The Effects of Childhood Abuse and Deprivation. New Haven, CT, Yale University Press, 1989, p 26

Strentz T: The Stockholm syndrome: law enforcement policy and hostage behavior, in Victims of Terrorism. Edited by Ochberg FM, Soskis DA. Boulder, CO, Westview, 1982, pp 149–163

Symonds M: Victim responses to terror: understanding and treatment, in Victims of Terrorism. Edited by Ochberg FM, Soskis DA. Boulder, CO, Westview, 1982, pp 95–103

Tennant CC, Goulston KJ, Dent OF: The psychological effects of being a prisoner of war: forty years after release. Am J Psychiatry 143:618–622, 1986

Timerman J: Prisoner Without a Name: Cell Without a Number (1980). Translated by Talbot T. New York, Vintage, 1988

van der Kolk BA: Compulsion to repeat the trauma: re-enactment, revictimization, and masochism. Psychiatr Clin North Am 12:389–411, 1989

van der Ploerd HM: Being held hostage in the Netherlands: a study of long-term aftereffects. Journal of Traumatic Stress 2:153–170, 1989

Walker L: The Battered Woman. New York, Harper & Row, 1979

Weschler L: Testimony of Mauricio Rosencof in The Great Exception: I: Liberty. New Yorker, April 3, 1989, pp 81–82

Wiesel E: Night. Translated by Rodway S. New York, Hill and Wang, 1960

Zanarini M, Gunderson J, Frakenburg F, et al: Discriminating borderline personality disorder from other Axis II disorders. Am J Psychiatry 147:161–167, 1990

# Epilogue

**Jonathan R. T. Davidson, M.D.**
**Edna B. Foa, Ph.D.**

These assembled chapters, arising from the DSM-IV process, have spotlighted a number of important topics in psychotraumatology. What do they teach us? How do they further our understanding of posttrauma psychopathology? What future directions do they suggest?

March (Chapter 3) and Kilpatrick and Resnick (Chapter 7) address the most distinctive feature of posttraumatic stress disorder (PTSD), the trauma, and lead us to consider the relationship between the traumatic event and development of PTSD. Quite clearly there is a dose-effect relationship in which the risk of developing PTSD increases with intensity and duration of the trauma. In this sense, we can view the relationship between trauma and the risk of PTSD as a continuum. However, we cannot disregard the modifying effects of predisposing vulnerability factors ("internal" factors) on this relationship. These factors include the following:

1. Genetic vulnerability to psychopathology in general, or to specific psychological disorders in particular;
2. Early adverse or traumatic experiences;
3. Personality characteristics (in particular, borderline, sociopathic, dependent, paranoid features, or neuroticism);
4. Recent life stresses or life change;
5. Deficient support systems;
6. Recent heavy use of alcohol; and
7. Locus of control (internal versus external) and pervasive sense of uncontrollability over stressful events.

We propose a model (Figure E–1) in which, as described above, the risk of developing PTSD is seen as a function both of the trauma ("external" factors) and of the victim ("internal" factors). We believe such an interactive model might have considerable heuristic benefit. Chronic PTSD can develop at any point in time, but commonly within 3 months, following a traumatic event. The likelihood (risk) of developing PTSD is partly determined by the severity and qualitative characteristics of the trauma on the one hand and by the victim's predisposing features on the other. Certain extreme traumatic events, above a given severity threshold, are likely to induce PTSD (at least initially) in most individuals, regardless of predisposition. At the opposite end, events that are minimally stressful to most people ("low-magnitude" events) could be traumatic in the presence of multiple predisposing factors. Moreover, we would posit that not all low-magnitude events can, indiscriminately, give rise to PTSD; more likely these events would contain certain qualitative elements common to higher magnitude events, or possibly activate older, dormant, traumatic experiences. In other words, the difference is one of degree rather than type. Most instances of PTSD will follow an event that is neither low magnitude nor of extreme magnitude and will be mediated by both external and internal factors.

In Chapter 2, Rothbaum and Foa have drawn attention to two questions that will surely produce further debate. First, they note that the great majority of rape victims in their study developed the DSM-III-R criteria for PTSD within the first 3 months after the rape. Does this mean that such a

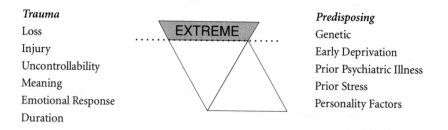

Below a certain threshold of trauma intensity, risk of developing PTSD is related to the sum of trauma severity and predisposition. A lesser effect from one factor is compensated for by a greater contribution from the other. Above a certain level of trauma severity, predisposing factors are not necessary.

**Figure E–1.**   Interactive and threshold determining effects of trauma and predisposition on development of PTSD.

response is normal? We must distinguish between statistical and clinical normality. We cannot consider PTSD symptoms to be normal reactions just because they are very common in some communities following disaster. By analogy, few would argue that dehydration or cholera are normal reactions because they may be widespread after normal disaster. Even if acute PTSD is common, it will remain a clinically abnormal or "meaningful" state. Awareness as to the high frequency of this reaction may lead to more vigorous preventative programs and/or public campaigning. Also, as Blank points out in Chapter 1, to acknowledge a brief PTSD in the individual's history can serve as useful alerting factor later on.

The second, and related, issue brought up by Rothbaum and Foa is that natural remission occurs within 3 months in more than half of all acute PTSD cases following rape. Does this mean that in some instances it is best not to intervene until a given period of time has passed? How would such a decision be made? If it was decided that crisis intervention/supportive counseling should be made available to all survivors in the immediate aftermath of trauma, then there would be a need to increase the provision of treatment resources, which at this time are grossly inadequate. Also, short-term intervention techniques would need to be developed, and their efficacy would need to be evaluated. The benefit of a 9-week course of treatment for rape victims with PTSD has already been demonstrated by Foa and colleagues (in press). Increased funding would be needed to implement such programs in training centers. One effect of our growing awareness, nevertheless, has already been the emergence of trauma-response counseling teams in the wake of natural disasters and acts of community violence, suggesting that we are now seeing a much needed societal response to this pressing problem.

In reviewing the epidemiology of PTSD, Davidson and Fairbank (Chapter 8) clearly demonstrate that the disorder occurs in a significant proportion of the population, being one of the more common preventable psychiatric disorders. If a sufficiently sensitive assessment procedure is used, the lifetime prevalence of PTSD in young American adults is 9%; the addition of subclinical posttraumatic syndromes brings this figure to 15%, or one in seven American citizens. Epidemiological studies are sorely needed, and one task must be for them to survey for exposure to trauma in the population, including a broad range of specific traumatic events. Risk factors for exposure to trauma may then be ascertained. Similarly, risk factors for the development of PTSD following exposure to traumatic events need be further studied. It would be important for such projects to enquire into cognitive and affective responses to the trauma, as well as to properties of the event itself. A comprehensive interview of this type should enquire about each trauma carefully. Such a labor-intensive procedure demands more than the usual amount of the interviewer-respondent rapport. Because such studies are of the greatest importance, it is hoped that investigators will not shirk from the task.

Several contributors have addressed the clinical and phenomenological aspects of PTSD. In his scholarly review, Blank identifies a complex course of the disorder, as well as the likely existence of different subtypes. These important observations may be profitably shared with patients and their relatives so that they might achieve a more realistic and informed expectation as to the course of this disorder. Perhaps the most compelling reason for introducing subtypes into a classification system of disorders is because of differential treatment responses. Certainly in the case of PTSD, the acute forms more urgently call for rapid treatment intervention, often utilizing abreactive, sedative, or crisis intervention techniques. Much more work needs to be accomplished in order to tease out the different indications for particular treatments, even to the point of drug selection and/or type of behavioral therapy used.

As noted in the Introduction, McNally's review of childhood PTSD (Chapter 4) along with the three reviews of PTSD in adult victim groups by Green, Keane, and Kilpatrick and Resnick (Chapters 5, 6, and 7, respectively), all agree with the basic construct validity and consistency of the criteria set. None of them points to the need for major changes in criteria. However, several of the symptoms are nonspecific to PTSD, being found in depression and other anxiety disorders, such as generalized anxiety disorder (GAD). This overlap could lead to a spurious comorbidity of the disorders.

As we noted in the Introduction, all three reviews of the PTSD adult groups express unhappiness with the requirement for three avoidant symptoms. It appears likely that many people with otherwise genuine PTSD symptoms are disenfranchised from the diagnosis, because they do not have the required three avoidant symptoms. Would the cause of PTSD be better served if only one or two avoidant criteria were required (i.e., avoidance of thoughts or feelings, avoidance of activity or situations that arouse recollection of the trauma)? A problem of boundary arises here, because these symptoms define simple phobias. A more general problem arises from the fact that the avoidance criteria include both phobic avoidance and dissociative-type symptoms, the combination of which seem to characterize PTSD and distinguish it from phobias. Should one phobic-avoidant symptom and one dissociative-avoidant symptom be set as a minimal requirement?

In his review of childhood PTSD, McNally makes the interesting observation that the relationship between incest and PTSD is inconsistent. This observation points out to the need for further inquiry into the matter, because Davidson and Smith (1990) have found incest to be the one trauma that invariably gives rise to PTSD in adult psychiatric patients.

Pitman's review (Chapter 9) provides evidence that patients with PTSD differ biologically in important ways from other individuals with anxiety disorders. It also poses the following question: How strong of an etiological effect must a pathogenic agent have, and how well understood must its mechanism be, in order to warrant elevating the resultant disease into a specific etiologically based category? Pitman encourages us to think about how we classify diseases. With our current ignorance about the etiology of PTSD, we can be spurred on to study those characteristics of the trauma and the individual that determine whether a person yields to, or is protected against, PTSD. Some work in this direction has already begun (e.g., D. S. Riggs, E. B. Foa, B. O. Rothbaum, unpublished data, 1991).

In Brett's review (Chapter 10), three options are proposed for the placement of PTSD, all of which have some merit. However, the evidence for regarding PTSD as a dissociative disease is the weakest. Reclassification of PTSD on the basis of etiology is not without its problems, but it would give to trauma the diagnostic prominence that many people think it deserves. We contend, and the epidemiological literature supports this contention, that traumatic events do not serve as nonspecific stressors for most psychiatric disorders; rather, they act specifically to increase the risk of a limited number of disorders, of which PTSD is one.

Herman's proposal for a new trauma-related disorder immediately raises the question of validation (Chapter 12). In contemplating the establishment of a new psychiatric disorder, one would do well to remember the maxims by which disorder categorization is supported. These include evidence of distinct symptomatology, well-delineated boundaries with regard to neighboring disorders, characteristic course, particular family patterns, unique pathophysiology, and distinctive treatment response. Data of this kind are needed to advance the field. The chapter by McNally and Saigh (Chapter 11) begins an attempt in this respect.

There is growing recognition that, in all probability, more than one form of abnormal posttraumatic stress reaction exists. In point of fact, DSM-III-R already acknowledges eight such disorders, which are scattered throughout the nomenclature. These disorders, listed in Table E–1, include brief reactive psychosis, dream anxiety disorders, conversion and somatization disorders, multiple personality disorder, and some types of borderline personality disorder. Adjustment disorder, while defined as being stress-induced, bears an unclear relation to traumatic, or extreme, stress. Among the proposed or potential new forms of posttraumatic disorders are Disorder of Extreme Stress Not Otherwise Specified (DESNOS), as described by Herman. To this, the epidemiological review by Davidson and Fairbank (Chapter 8) suggests for possible consideration a posttraumatic form of depression, which seems to differ in important ways from nontraumatic primary depression. A concerted research effort is needed to apply common

Table E–1.    DSM-III-R disorders that may be caused by trauma

| DSM-III-R Disorder | Importance of Trauma as Being Necessary[a] |
|---|---|
| Posttraumatic Stress Disorder | +++++ |
| Brief Reactive Psychosis | +++++ |
| Multiple Personality Disorder | +++++ |
| Psychogenic Fugue | ++++ |
| Psychogenic Amnesia | ++++ |
| Depersonalization Disorder | +++ |
| Conversion Disorder | +++ |
| Dream Anxiety Disorder | +++ |
| Borderline Personality Disorder | +++ |
| Antisocial Personality Disorder | ++ |
| Somatization Disorder | ++ |
| Simple Phobia | + |
| [Adjustment Disorder | Unclear] |
| **Potential Disorders** | |
| Disorder of Extreme Stress NOS | +++++ |
| Posttraumatic Depression | +++++ |

[a]This column provides an estimate, based on the DSM-III-R text, as to the importance of trauma (or severe stress) as a necessary factor (i.e., it represents the extent to which the occurrence of trauma is a sine qua non for the disorder). An arbitrary rating of +++++ has been assigned to PTSD.

methods to study all those psychological disorders in which the original occurrence of trauma served as a necessary (i.e., etiological) factor.

Insofar as most psychiatric disorder is related to "stress," one critical issue remains: How we can agree on distinguishing traumatic from nontraumatic stress? Some of our contributors (e.g., March [Chapter 3] and Kilpatrick and Resnick [Chapter 7]) provide guidelines in this respect, suggesting crucial factors of the event or of the victim's perception and appraisal of it. Further empirical support of the role of victim perception in PTSD has been provided by Riggs and colleagues (D. S. Riggs, E. B. Foa, B. O. Rothbaum, unpublished data, 1991).

In summary, PTSD presents one of the largest clinical, research, and societal challenges of all psychiatric disorders. Clinical researchers and policy makers in the field of psychological trauma are to be commended for having achieved so much in so short a period of time; the courage of trauma survivors and their supporters is to be commended, because they too have contributed in important ways toward the furtherance of knowledge. However, many tasks lie ahead, and we hope the reviews presented in this book will have contributed toward this end.

# References

Davidson JRT, Smith RD: Traumatic experiences in psychiatric outpatients. Journal of Traumatic Stress 3:459–474, 1990

Foa EB, Rothbaum BO, Riggs D, et al: Treatment of posttraumatic stress disorder in rape victims. J Consult Clin Psychol (in press)

# Appendix 1

# Suggested Recommendations for DSM-IV on Course and Subtypes

**Arthur S. Blank, M.D.**

## Recommended Description of Course

**Course.**    The course of posttraumatic stress disorder (PTSD) varies considerably and may be influenced by duration, severity, and complexity of trauma; personality, social supports and other intervening variables posttrauma; plus other factors. Acute PTSD is specified when the onset occurs between 1 and 12 months of traumatically stressful events, and delayed type when the onset is after 12 months posttrauma. Either acute or delayed PTSD may progress to chronic PTSD, which should be specified when diagnostic requirements have been met for a period of more than 1 year. Within 1 month after experiencing a traumatically stressful event, the V code "Uncomplicated posttraumatic stress reaction" should be used. Over time, PTSD symptoms may wax and wane, justifying use of the modifiers "recurrent" or "residual." "Recurrent" should be specified when fully-diagnosable PTSD has returned after an interval of no or few symptoms. "Residual" PTSD may be used where diagnostic criteria have been fully met in the past, and symptoms are currently below threshold (e.g., during a phase when diagnostic requirements are met for one or two but not all three of Criteria B, C, and D, following a phase when diagnostic requirements were fully met).

237

In the individual case, the relative predominance of intrusion, avoidance, and hyperarousal symptoms may vary over time.

## Recommended Text for V Code

V xx.xx *Uncomplicated posttraumatic stress reaction to traumatic stress,* such as disaster, criminal assault, wartime combat, or other similar traumatic stress. The various symptoms seen in posttraumatic stress disorder are also seen in individuals who have experienced traumatic stressors but where there are significantly fewer symptoms, and also possibly of less variety, than is the case in PTSD. Especially during the first year after a traumatic stress experience, these symptoms are common, and may not add up to the diagnostic requirements for PTSD. Such symptoms may disappear with time, or may attenuate with time while persisting to some degree for years, at least episodically. Often persons with a few posttraumatic symptoms (e.g., war veterans), who do not show full-blown PTSD, regard such symptoms as normal. This code should also be used for cases where 1 month has not yet elapsed since the experiencing of traumatic stressors.

## Additional Recommendations

The requirement for 1-month duration (as distinguished from 1 month's time elapsed since experiencing the traumatically stressful events), present in DSM-III-R (page 251), should be dropped. There is no evidence that PTSD is the less so for being brief; and the documentation of a brief episode in a patient's history may serve a useful alerting function in the event of recurrent symptoms at some future date, particularly given continuing difficulties in recognizing the disorder clinically. Rather, it is recommended that the E criterion be revised as follows: "A minimum of 1 month has elapsed since the experiencing of traumatic stressor(s)."

## Comments

It will be very useful clinically to provide guidance concerning use of the terms acute, chronic, delayed, residual, and recurrent as indicated previously, accompanied by the suggested language that informs clinicians that the course of PTSD can be highly varied. Awareness that PTSD may recede with time promotes therapeutic optimism, which is sometimes helpful; awareness that PTSD may recur may prevent some clinicians and patients from experiencing undue discouragement. Articulating the realities of residual PTSD and V code-type symptoms will enhance understanding of the fact that posttrauma symptoms often work out and are ameliorated gradually over time.

It is especially important to note that the onset of PTSD can be delayed, as was done in DSM-III-R, and to amplify that point slightly more than did DSM-III-R, as recommended here. This will mitigate against some clinicians' tendency to miss PTSD when a longer time interval has elapsed between the stressful events and the onset of diagnosable PTSD.

It appears most appropriate to avoid designating as *types or subtypes*, the longitudinal course qualifiers of acute, chronic, delayed, recurrent, and residual, in line with the practice in DSM-III-R of reserving the designations of type of subtype for forms of a disorder that are distinctly different in severity or symptom pattern (e.g., the various types of schizophrenia or depressive disorder). "Course" and "subtypes" were, it appears in retrospect, somewhat inappropriately lumped together in DSM-III-R. The longitudinal course qualifiers recommended here refer simply to variations on the time axis (i.e., onset, duration, and waxing and waning of symptoms) and do not reflect major differences in symptom constellation, insofar as is known at present.

# Appendix 2

# Suggested Recommendations for DSM-IV: Duration, Subtypes, and Posttraumatic Stress Disorder In Relation to Adjustment Disorder

Barbara Olasov Rothbaum, Ph.D.
Edna B. Foa, Ph.D.

### Retain a Duration Requirement

However, a 1-month duration of symptoms for a diagnosis of posttraumatic stress disorder (PTSD) is inadequate. We propose a 3-month duration requirement instead, implying a chronic disorder.

### Do Not Include Subtypes

The DSM-III distinctions of acute versus chronic or delayed PTSD are not supported by empirical evidence. Delayed PTSD should be discussed in the text but should not be regarded as a subtype.

### Adjustment Disorder is Not an Appropriate Interim Diagnosis

Severe reactions within the first 3 months posttrauma ideally can be considered as posttraumatic stress reaction, a V code diagnosis.

# Appendix 3

# A Description of the Posttraumatic Stress Disorder Field Trial

Dean G. Kilpatrick, Ph.D.
Heidi S. Resnick, Ph.D.

## Overview

Currently, a Field Trial Study is being conducted to examine possible changes in PTSD Criterion A as well as other questions raised by the DSM-IV PTSD Committee. The principal investigators are Dean Kilpatrick, Ph.D., and Bessel van der Kolk, M.D. Other investigators involved in conducting the study at 5 sites across the country include David Pelcovitz, Ph.D., Patricia Resick, Ph.D., Heidi Resnick, Ph.D., and Susan Roth, Ph.D. The final section of this appendix includes sections of the Field Trial Proposal, "An Empirical Evaluation of Criterion A in Posttraumatic Stress Disorder," that specifically relate to an examination of the impact of proposed changes in Criterion A on PTSD symptoms as measured by Criteria B, C, D, and E.

## An Empirical Evaluation of Criterion A in Posttraumatic Stress Disorder

### Specific Aims

The major goal of the proposed field trial is to gather empirical data about the impact of alternative versions of Criterion A, the stressor criterion, on the likelihood of obtaining a PTSD diagnosis as measured by Criteria B, C, D, and E. Clearly, Criterion A plays a key gatekeeping function in the diagnosis of PTSD, because it identifies types of potentially stressful events and experiences that render an individual either eligible or ineligible to be evaluated for PTSD using the remaining diagnostic criteria. It follows that the prevalence of PTSD should vary substantially depending on the breadth of potentially stressful events that are included in Criterion A. Several types of potentially distressing events are specifically excluded from Criterion A in the DSM-III-R (American Psychiatric Association 1987) text (i.e., simple bereavement, chronic illness, severe financial losses, or serious marital conflict). One major criticism of the current DSM-III-R definition of Criterion A is that some of these excluded events appear to produce symptoms in the B, C, and D criteria that are virtually identical to PTSD symptoms experienced by people whose stressors are included in Criterion A. A second criticism is that the Criterion A requirement that stressor events be "outside the range of usual human experience and that would be markedly distressing to almost anybody" requires normative information about the prevalence of stressor events and about how distressing most people find them that is not available to assessing clinicians or researchers. A third criticism is that there are substantial differences between the DSM-III-R and the proposed *International Classification of Diseases, 10th Revision* (ICD-10) definition of Criterion A (see Table A–1).

Whereas the DSM-IV PTSD Advisory Committee is in virtual agreement that some change in Criterion A is necessary, suggested changes range from totally eliminating Criterion A to making modest revisions. However, a majority of the Committee appears to support a revision that would emphasize not only the stressor event but also the individual's cognitive appraisal of, or subjective distress in response to, that event (see draft definition in Table A–1). Given this new emphasis on cognitive appraisal and reactions of intense fear, distress, or helplessness as factors that might product PTSD, it is clear that stressors other than the typical "high-magnitude" stressors now included in Criterion A might be so cognitively appraised by some individuals and/or be associated with intense physical and emotional reactions, and therefore, be capable of producing PTSD symptoms. Thus, it is essential to collect data on low- as well as high-magnitude stressors, patient's cognitive appraisals, and initial physical and emotional reactions to those events, and to examine for potential stressor event–person interactions with respect to PTSD likelihood. Collecting such data is the major focus of this field trial.

Empirical examination of the impact of various proposed changes in Criterion A can best be accomplished by a field trial that includes the following assessment procedure.

1. An independent assessment of stressors, or potentially traumatic events, must be conducted with each patient. Events assessed must include the "low-magnitude" stressors currently excluded from Criterion A as well as the "high-magnitude" stressors that are included in Criterion A. In addition, as part of the trauma history, within-event exposure charac-

---

Table A–1.   Definitions of stressor criterion for PTSD diagnosis in DSM-III, DSM-III-R, ICD-10

---

**DSM-III CRITERION A**

Existence of a recognizable stressor that would evoke significant symptoms of distress in almost everyone.

**DSM-III-R CRITERION A**

The person has experienced an event that is outside the range of usual human experience and that would be markedly distressing to almost anyone, e.g., serious threat to one's life or physical integrity; serious threat or harm to one's children, spouse, or other close relatives and friends; sudden destruction of one's home or community; or seeing another person who has recently been, or is being, seriously injured or killed as the result of an accident or physical violence.

**ICD-10 CRITERION A**

Exposure to an exceptional mental or physical stressor, either brief or prolonged.

**PROPOSED DSM-IV CRITERION A**

**Alternative One**

The person has experienced, witnessed, or been confronted with an event or events which involve actual or threatened death or injury, or a threat to the physical integrity of oneself or others.

**Alternative Two**

A1  The person has experienced, witnessed, or learned about an event or events which involve actual or threatened death or injury, or a threat to the physical integrity of oneself or others.

A2  The person's response involved intense fear, distress, helplessness or horror.

**Alternative Three (ICD-10 Proposal)**

Exposure to an exceptional mental or physical stressor, either brief or prolonged.

Events commonly eliciting this response include military combat, sexual or other violent assault, human or natural disasters, and severe accidents. Infrequently, in the presence of heightened personal vulnerability, events that are objectively less threatening may induce the disorder.

teristics such as being injured, suffering bodily damage, or witnessing violence during an event should be assessed.

2. The patient's subjective cognitive, physiological, and affective reactions in response to each low- and high-magnitude stressor event experienced should be assessed along dimensions of fear, other distress, and/or helplessness.

3. PTSD symptoms measured by Criteria B, C, and D should be assessed independently using a multimethod procedure.

4. Those patients with PTSD as defined as meeting Criteria B, C, and D should be determined.

5. A multivariate analysis should be conducted with the PTSD-positive and PTSD-negative groups that examines whether the life history of the PTSD positive is more likely to include:
   a) high versus low magnitude stressors;
   b) cognitive appraisals of stressor events and initial physical and emotional reactions to events; or
   c) interactive effects between stressor magnitude and cognitive appraisal and/or initial subjective distress.

## Method

### Samples

Four samples will be assessed in the field trial:

1. 300 patients from five clinical treatment sites specializing in provision of mental health treatment to victims of high-magnitude stressors;

2. 100 nonpatients who had experienced high-magnitude stressors, recruited from the general population via use of random digit dial (RDD) telephone screening;

3. 100 nonpatients who had experienced low-magnitude stressors within the year prior to assessment, also recruited from the general population via RDD telephone screening; and

4. 100 patients seeking treatment for distress related to exposure to low magnitude stressors.

Those in the low-magnitude stressor groups must never have experienced a high-magnitude stressor. All participants must be at least 15 years old at the time of assessment. Because of the breadth of types of trauma victims treated at the clinical treatment sites, it is expected that the 300 members of the sample of patients exposed to high-magnitude stressors will have experienced a wide range of high-magnitude stressor events and that they will display an equally wide range of cognitive appraisals of those events. Importantly, some but not all of these patients would be expected to have PTSD as measured by Criteria B, C, and D. Likewise, the 100 members of the sample of patients exposed to low-magnitude stressors should vary with respect to type of stressor and cognitive appraisal.

The two nonpatient comparison groups will be identified and recruited by RDD telephone interviews. Briefly described, RDD is a sampling procedure that uses randomly generated telephone numbers to select households in a geographical area of interest. It covers about 96% of all households (the percentage of households with telephones) and includes nonlisted numbers. An eligible respondent is then randomly selected within each household and interviewed. Contrary to popular belief, it is possible to use RDD telephone interviewing to gather data about a host of sensitive topics and to achieve high response rates and considerable cooperation from respondents. For example, in an ongoing National Institute on Drug Abuse (NIDA)-funded project that is screening a national probability sample of 4,000 adult women for history of traumatic events (e.g., rape and homicide death of family members), substance abuse behavior, and PTSD, our research group is achieving an 85% response rate (Kilpatrick et al. 1989). The major advantage to use of RDD as a sampling, screening, and recruitment procedure is that the samples of individuals exposed to high- and low-magnitude stressors it will identify are much more likely to be representative of the general population than samples recruited via media or from patient groups.

### Assessment Measures

All 600 subjects will be assessed using each of the following measures:

1. *High-Magnitude Stressor Events Structured Interview:* This interview, to be administered by the research assistant, will screen for lifetime history of completed rape, other sexual assault, serious physical assault, other violent crime, homicide death of family members or close friends, serious accidents, natural or manmade disasters, or military combat. Data

will be gathered about each stressor with respect to its stressor dimensions (e.g., objective life threat, exposure to grotesquery in the form of dead bodies or body parts, extent of personal bereavement produced by stressor event, and extent of physical injuries sustained) and the patient's subjective cognitive appraisal of the event (e.g., perceived life threat, experience of fear and other distress, physical symptoms of panic during the event, attribution of helplessness and loss of control, and extent of unexpectedness of the stressor's onset).

2. *Low-Magnitude Stressor Events Structured Interview:* This will measure stress or events that are presently excluded from Criterion A (e.g., nonviolent death of family or friends, chronic illnesses, business losses, and marital or relationship conflicts) and that have occurred in the year prior to assessment. Each event will be rated by respondents along the same stressor and cognitive appraisal dimensions described above.

3. *Posttraumatic Stress Disorder Symptoms:* PTSD will be assessed using multiple methods. The primary method will be to use the PTSD module of the Structured Clinical Interview for DSM-III-R (SCID), which will be administered by a trained clinician. A portion of these interviews will be tape recorded and reviewed by another clinician to provide an estimate of interjudge reliability. A second method will be a modified version of the Diagnostic Interview Schedule (DIS; Robins et al. 1981) PTSD module that is being used in several epidemiological studies. This version does not require the patient to link symptoms with the traumatic event and gathers information about the content of intrusive symptoms. A third method will be the administration of three self-report scales: 1) the Impact of Event Scale (IES; Horowitz et al. 1979); 2) the Symptom Checklist 90-R (SCL-90-R, Derogatis 1977) and the recently developed Crime-Related PTSD Scale (Saunders et al. 1990) that was developed by selecting SCL-90-R items that best discriminated between PTSD positive and negative cases in a community sample, using an empirical criterion keying approach; and 3) the Civilian Mississippi PTSD Scale (Keane et al. 1988).

## Approach

The major focus of data analysis will be to determine how type of stressor (high versus low magnitude), within-event exposure characteristics, subjective cognitive appraisal and distress, and the stressor-cognitive appraisal/subjective distress interaction influence PTSD likelihood as measured by a consensus diagnosis based on Criteria B, C, and D. Analyses will be conducted using the dichotomous variables of full PTSD diagnosis, or individual B, C, or D criteria, as well as continuous measures of number of total PTSD symptoms, and numbers of individual criterion symptoms (i.e., total number of reexperiencing, avoidance, or increased arousal items). Several members of the Committee have suggested the utility of a strategy of working backward from the identification of the diagnosis or the pattern of symptomatic distress characteristic of PTSD, to the likelihood that the subject has been exposed to particular types of traumatic events (individual or multiple events). An exploratory canonical discriminant function or correlation analysis might allow for an identification of types or patterns of stressor events associated with particular symptom patterns.

At this time, there are few data available regarding the association between what we are labeling as low-magnitude stressors and PTSD as it is defined by Criteria B, C, and D. Therefore, the impact of broadening Criterion A to allow for stressor events that objectively appear to be less threatening, but are subjectively perceived as "traumatic" (i.e., extremely distressing, unexpected, or uncontrollable) by a subset of those who experience them, is unknown at this time.

A second set of analyses will focus on the sensitivity, specificity, positive predictive power, and negative predictive power of various PTSD measures using the consensus diagnosis as the criterion. This procedure was used in the National Vietnam Veterans Readjustment Study (NVVRS). In that study, multiple PTSD measures, including IES, Mississippi Scale, and SCID interview data, were employed to arrive at a "composite" diagnosis of current PTSD. Preliminary results of the NVVRS (Kulka et al. 1990) indicated that the DIS interview had high specificity in relation to the composite diagnosis of PTSD, but a low sensitivity rate. In the current study, the sensitivity and specificity rates of the nonclinician-administered modified DIS and the clinician-administered SCID interview schedules will be assessed in relation to a consensus diagnosis based on interview and self-report data.

# References

American Psychiatric Association: Diagnostic and Statistical Manual of Mental Disorders, 3rd Edition, Revised. Washington, DC, American Psychiatric Association, 1987

Derogatis LR: SCL-90: Administration, scoring & procedure manual-I for the R (revised) version. Baltimore, MD, Johns Hopkins University School of Medicine, 1977

Horowitz M, Wilner N, Alvarez W: Impact of Event Scale: Measure of subjective stress. Psychosom Med 41(3):209–218, 1979

Keane TM, Caddell JM, Taylor KL: The Mississippi scale for combat-related PTSD: studies in reliability and validity. J Consult Clin Psychology 56:85–90, 1988

Kilpatrick DG, Best CL, Lipovsky JA, et al: Risk factors for substance abuse: A longitudinal study. National Institute on Drug Abuse Grant No. DA 05220-01A2, 1989

Kulka RA, Schlenger WE, Fairbank JA, et al: Trauma and the Vietnam War Generation. New York, Brunner/Mazel, 1990

Robins LN, Helzer JE, Croughan J, et al: National Institute of Mental Health Diagnostic Interview Schedule: its history, characteristics, and validity. Arch Gen Psychiatry 38:381–389, 1981

Saunders BE, Mandoki KA, Kilpatrick DG: Development of a crime-related posttraumatic stress disorder scale within the Symptom Checklist-90-Revised. J Traumatic Stress 3:439–448, 1990

# Index

Page numbers in boldface refer to tables or figures.